THE DEVELOPMENT
AND MANAGEMENT
OF MEDICAL GROUPS

by
Gerald S. Benedict

THE DEVELOPMENT AND MANAGEMENT OF MEDICAL GROUPS

Author:
Gerald S. Benedict

Published by:
Medical Group Management Association
104 Inverness Terrace East
Englewood, CO 80112-5306
(303) 799-1111
and
American Medical Association
515 North State Street
Chicago, IL 60610
(312) 464-5000

Medical Group Management Association (MGMA) prints publications that are intended to provide current and accurate information and are designed to assist readers in becoming more familiar with the subject matter covered. Such publications are distributed with the understanding that MGMA does not render any legal, accounting or other professional advice. No representations or warranties are made concerning the application of legal or other principles discussed by the authors to any specific fact situation, nor is any prediction made concerning how any particular judge, government official or other person who will interpret or apply such principles. Specific factual situations should be discussed with professional advisors.

Copyright © 1996
Medical Group Management Association
104 Inverness Terrace East
Englewood, CO 80112-5306
(303) 799-1111

ISBN 1-56829-049-7

Acknowledgments

The Development and Management of Medical Groups is a synthesis of my experiences and ideas and those of colleagues too numerous to mention. Certain individuals deserve a special thank you for their contributions to this book: **C.V. Allen, M.D.** and **C.R. Maino, M.D.** of Gould Medical Group; **Debra Roth**, **John Ferguson** and **Cindy Zontek** of Gould Medical Foundation; **Sue Cejka** of Cejka and Company; **Nancy Severson** of Lutheran Medical Center; **Joe and Marilyn Davis** of Medimetrix Group; **Tom Mayer, M.D.** of Strategic Healthcare Management, and **Rick Wesslund** of BDC Advisors.

Fred E. Graham II, Ph.D., FACMPE, CAE, Senior Vice President/COO, **Dennis L. Barnhardt, APR**, Director of Communications, **Barbara Hamilton**, Library Resource Center Director, and **Stephanie Wyllyamz**, Communications Specialist, of Medical Group Management Association provided valuable assistance in the publication process.

I would also like to thank my wife Nancy, and my parents Jim and Muriel, for their support and encouragement during this project.

About the Author

A principal with Medimetrix Group, a national healthcare consulting firm, Gerald Benedict has over 20 years of experience in public accounting, healthcare consulting, hospital and group practice administration and group practice development.

Benedict provides Medimetrix Group with firm-wide leadership in the development and implementation of physician group practices, management services organizations, physician/hospital organizations and integrated delivery systems.

Prior to joining Medimetrix, Benedict was president and chief executive officer of Community Health Services Organization, an affiliate of Denver's Lutheran Medical Center. In that position, he directed all of Lutheran's managed care contracting and operations, ambulatory services and physician support services. He was also responsible for leading the development of Lutheran's ambulatory care and physician integration strategies.

The author also spent eight years at Gould Medical Foundation, a large, capitated, multispecialty medical clinic in California, where he served as president and chief executive officer. During his tenure at Gould Medical Foundation, he was directly responsible for converting Gould from a for-profit medical group into one of the first not-for-profit, tax-exempt medical foundations in California. He successfully affiliated the Foundation with Sutter Health Systems of Sacramento, Calif. He has also served as a director with BDC Advisors, a nationally known consulting firm and as a partner in two CPA firms.

Benedict is a frequent national and regional speaker and is a member of Medical Group Management Association, the Healthcare Financial Management Association and the American Institute of Certified Public Accountants. He resides with his wife, Nancy, in Denver, Colo.

Table of Contents

Part II — The Management of Medical Groups

Table of Charts

Chapter Three

Chapter Four

Chapter Five

Foreword

The American physician practice environment has evolved in the 20th century from the days of the general practitioner making house calls to one with varied physician practice alternatives. Physicians today can choose from many options: (1) solo practice, (2) affiliations with other independent practitioners for joint access to management services or managed care contracts, (3) ownership and/or employment in single-specialty or multispecialty groups, and (4) affiliation, alignment or employment with hospitals, health plans, or others in local, regional, or national health systems. The transition to these sophisticated delivery systems has been stimulated by several forces in the health care industry, with a predominant one being the rise of managed care. In the last few years, the health care payment system has become more complex while demands of all health care consumers have risen. The ability of physicians to thrive financially, especially in solo practice, has become more difficult.

With the business of delivering health care becoming increasingly complicated and competitive, many physicians look to medical groups for salvation. As they transition from solo practice or medical schools to medical groups, little information is available on the potential rewards and pitfalls that lie ahead. When physicians (and other interested parties) start down the medical group path, it is comforting to know that others have blazed the trail. The real life experiences of physicians, administrators, consultants and others who develop and manage medical groups throughout this country are summarized in the following pages. It is hoped that their experiences will help current and future medical group leaders achieve success.

PART ONE

The Development of Medical Groups

The development of medical groups has been accelerating throughout the second half of the 20th century. "Group physicians, who were only 1.2 percent of the profession in 1940, rose to 2.6 percent in 1946, 5.2 percent in 1959 and 12.8 percent by 1969 ... By 1980 the 88,000 doctors in groups represented a quarter of the doctors in active practice."[1]

Preliminary data from the American Medical Association (AMA) Census of Medical Groups for 1995 indicates that there are approximately 19,200 groups, representing about 223,000, or one-third of, physicians. The average size of all groups is 11.8 physicians. The average size of single specialty groups is six physicians, while the average size of multispecialty groups is 26 physicians. There is no question that group practice is becoming more prevalent; the number of groups is increasing every year.[2]

Recent graduates from medical school are even more likely than established physicians to practice in a medical group. According to the Cambridge Management Group, Inc., 75 percent of the medical school graduates in 1993 indicated a preference to practice in a group practice setting, with an even higher percentage of female residents expressing this preference.[3] A 1990 survey conducted by the Association of American Medical Colleges showed that only 2.9 percent of medical students plan to enter solo practice. Among the students indicating preference for a private clinical practice career path, 66.7 percent indicated a preference for group practice.[4]

What is fueling the development of medical groups? Is the solo physician practice becoming extinct? Will physicians become assembly-line workers in someone else's business? What will happen to the physician-patient relationship? As market forces shape health care, will quality care and personal service be sacrificed in the name of efficiency and low cost?

Health care consumers, physicians and other providers are very concerned about the answers to these questions. The traditional profession of medicine is at risk. Patients are being denied access to their longtime personal physicians by managed care plans while the number of uninsured reaches catastrophic levels (41 million Americans, or 16.1 percent of the population, had no health insurance in 1993).[5] There is a consensus that the health care system in this country is broken (without any consensus on the right solutions, or the right way to implement national health care reform).

Physicians are becoming increasingly disenchanted by the hassles of solo practice and the new "rules of the game." Many physicians are joining or forming medical groups (or others are "buying their practices" and organizing them into groups) to maintain some control and influence over the forces shaping their futures. Other physicians are still in the "denial" or "anger" stages and refusing to "join the crowd" in medical groups. Some are just hanging on to solo practice until they can retire. Physicians leaving urban centers and moving to rural areas are shocked to find out that the "good old days" are already gone.

How did the medical group movement get started in this country? What are the forces driving physicians to join medical groups? Do medical groups provide benefits for physicians and health care consumers? What are the steps required to form and implement medical groups? The following discussion attempts to answer these questions as well as demonstrate why properly structured and governed medical groups are well positioned to serve the needs of their communities in the new health care environment.

Notes

1 The *Social Transformation of American Medicine*, Paul Starr, 1982, p. 425.

2 *Medical Groups in the U.S.*, 1995 Edition, American Medical Association, Chicago, Ill., p. 1.

3 Cambridge Management Group, Inc., Cambridge, Mass., 1994.

4 *The Journal of Ambulatory Care Management: Physician Practice*, Editors I. Blumstein, MBA and M. Tosos, MSBA, CPA, 1992.

5 "43% of Noncitizens Lack Health Care, Study Group Reports," *New York Times*, Jan. 24, 1995.

CHAPTER ONE

Historical Background

What is a medical group?

One source of confusion, even within the medical field, is a common definition of a medical group. For this discussion, a medical group refers to an organization of physicians with actual economic practice integration. Preferred provider organizations (PPOs), independent practice associations (IPAs) and physician hospital organizations (PHOs) — ways physicians are organizing for managed care contracting — are not considered medical groups since most physician members of PPOs, IPAs and PHOs do not economically integrate their practices. Staff models, where physicians are direct employees of health plans, health systems or others, are also not included in this discussion as medical groups. The American Medical Association and the Medical Group Management Association define medical group practice as:

> The provision of health care services by three or more physicians who are formally organized as a legal entity in which business and clinical facilities, records and personnel are shared. Income from medical services provided by the group are treated as receipts of the group and distributed according to some prearranged plan.[1]

A successful medical group is, however, more than just an economic device. As stated by Russell Lee, M.D., founder of the prestigious Palo Alto Medical Clinic in Northern California:

> Group practice is a way of life ... it is more than an arrangement for the convenience of physicians ... Properly conceived and properly practiced, it provides the most efficient means of bringing the diverse skills and achievements of modern medicine to those who need help. It provides a climate in which can thrive the finest relationship between doctors, a relationship which brings together various specialists to devote all of their skills to the ame-

lioration of human ills ... It provides an atmosphere of mutual helpfulness ... It gives the doctor a sense of security ... from the feeling that he belongs to a group which ... supports and comforts ... A proper group is like a proper family ... one belongs.[2]

Origins of medical groups

Medical groups are fairly recent phenomenons. The modern day medical group is rooted in the latter part of the last century. Some of the medical groups formed in the 19th century still exist in a number of forms, and others have disappeared. Specialization led physicians to group together for the practice of medicine in the late 19th century. It forced itself on the medical profession for reasons of sheer technological complexity. With the advent and growth of specialization, it became necessary to find methods to make it acceptable. One of these methods was group practice.[3]

Another factor in the origins of medical groups was the organization of physician faculties by medical schools. One of the earliest of these was Johns Hopkins University, whose funds and prestige were instrumental in forming an outstanding faculty medical group.

The Mayo Clinic

Among the many physicians who visited the Johns Hopkins University Group to learn and observe were two young surgeons who had recently joined their father in practice in Rochester, Minn. They were Charles and William Mayo, and their subsequent establishment of the Mayo Clinic influenced medical group development in the 20th century in a major way.

The Mayo brothers developed, crystallized and publicized the idea of the medical group. No history of group practice would be of value if it failed to recognize the tremendous part played by the Mayos. From 1883, when the elder son joined his father in practice, until 1900, when the group had grown to seven or eight staff members, the Mayo group was probably considered a projection of individual practice. This setup was changed by the addition of Dr. Henry Plummer to the staff. As exceptional as the brothers, he introduced laboratory and X-ray services and formed the nucleus for a medical department. During the first decade of the century, the Mayo Clinic gained national and international fame. In the same era, other groups were founded, many of them by former Mayo assistants or Fellows.[4] By 1914, the Mayo Clinic included 17 doctors on its staff. By 1929, when the Mayo Clinic was housed in its own 15-story building, that figure had grown to 386 physicians and dentists, backed by 895 staff members.[5]

Paul Starr, the Pulitzer Prize-winning author of the history of American medicine, describes the development of the Mayo Clinic:

> The point of origin for group practice in America was the Mayo Clinic ... the two brothers increasingly specialized in surgery, adopting the newest techniques and creatively extending them in new operations ... Their reputation for skill, invention and exceedingly low mortality rates attracted both patients and respect ... they decided to expand partly because they wanted to travel to the East and Europe to keep up with new scientific developments.
>
> Over the next 10 years, they added several younger doctors who were adept in new diagnostic techniques, such as blood tests, X-rays and bacteriological examinations ... The specialization in diagnostic techniques reflected both the tremendous scientific advances in diagnosis and the distinctive needs of the enterprise ...
>
> Diagnostic work and research gradually became as important as surgery ... The clinic also developed into a center of graduate medical education, augmenting its influence in the profession ...
>
> From Rochester, the admirers of the Mayo Clinic spread out across the country ... A young doctor who worked as an assistant at the clinic from 1906 to 1909, Donald Guthrie, founded the Guthrie Clinic in Sayre, Penn., in 1910. In the summer of 1908, a general practitioner from Topeka, Kan., Charles F. Menninger ... is said to have declared, I have been to the Mayos and I have seen a great thing ... we are going to have a clinic like that right here in Topeka.[6]

The early 20th century

Several modern-day American medical groups had their genesis in the early part of this century. An American Medical Association (AMA) survey conducted in 1932 found that, of existing groups, 18 had been founded prior to 1912. In that year another nine were established. The period from 1914 to 1920 saw a high rate of growth with a peak from 1918 to 1920. As of 1932, the AMA found about 300 group practices with a median size of between five and six physicians. In another survey published in 1932, C. Rufus Rorem estimated there were about 150 private group clinics in the United States, involving about 1,500 to 2,000 physicians.[7] World War II provided a major stimulus to formation and growth of medical groups. Prior to this war, the military services had virtually ignored specialization among physicians. Wartime reorganization of large military units resulted in a clinic-type operation. So many physicians were impressed by the advantages gained that a survey conducted by the American Medical Association during the war revealed that more than 50 percent of physicians in the service hoped to enter group practice on their return to civilian practice. The immediate postwar years saw a great increase in group practice.[8]

Most of the medical groups formed in the early 20th century were located in rural areas. A 1933 AMA survey found half of the medical groups in cities with less than 25,000 people, and two thirds in cities with less than 50,000. Only 4 percent of the groups were located in cities with a population of more than half a million. These findings contradict the usual expectation that complex organizations develop first and rapidly in urban areas. The absence of large voluntary hospitals in small cities created an opportunity in the early 1900s for the development of proprietary clinics. Similarly, the 1933 AMA study pointed out that, in large cities with ample hospitals and laboratory services, doctors did not have the same motive for forming groups. The available hospital and outpatient facilities provided medical care for many who, in a smaller place, would patronize a group.[9]

Prepaid medical groups

Another chapter in the history of medical groups began with the development of prepaid medical groups (payment for medical services made in advance and based on a set fee), highlighted by the 1933 formation of Kaiser Permanente. *The Story of the Permanente Medical Group* describes how the founding physician of the Kaiser Permanente medical group, Dr. Sidney Garfield, learned how group practice might work while serving as a surgical resident at Los Angeles County Hospital:

> "Sidney Garfield ... formed a close friendship with two residents in internal medicine ... [they] shared with each other the fascinating clinical experiences of Los Angeles County Hospital. They referred cases back and forth to each other and, over a period of time, developed a collegiality that would last for a lifetime ... Playing together, learning from each other, they acquired their medical skills in a socially responsible hospital setting where patients were treated without consideration of payment."[10]

Later, when Dr. Garfield owned a small hospital in the Southern California desert, he agreed to take prepayment for medical services.

> Henry J. Kaiser ... had been impressed by the program Dr. Sidney Garfield set up for his workers ... The industrialist decided to carry over the same practice of providing comprehensive health

services to workers in his shipyards and steel mills on the West Coast, even though they were in closer proximity to urban medical resources ... Because of the war, local hospitals and physicians were considerably overburdened and offered little opposition. In 1942 Kaiser set up two Permanente Foundations to run the medical programs — one for the Vancouver-Portland region, the other for his workers in Richmond and Fontana, Calif. At their zenith, these programs covered about 200,000 people, but as the war ended, the work force declined precipitously. The plans were almost closed when in late 1945 the decision was made to open them to the public. With an almost missionary zeal, Henry Kaiser believed he could reorganize medical care on a self-sufficient basis, independent of government, to provide millions of Americans with prepaid and comprehensive services at prices they could afford. Ten years after the war, the Kaiser Permanente health plan had a growing network of hospitals and clinics and a half million people enrolled ... The appeal of these prepayment plans originally had little to do with any price advantage in their premiums. Indeed, their premiums were usually more expensive than insurance. However, their coverage was also more comprehensive. When compared to indemnity or service-benefit plans, they had relatively few exclusions, limits or copayments ... The prepaid group practice plans, moreover, offered service of apparently high quality, partly because of the advantages of group practice, such as easier consultation among specialists as well as the greater emphasis on preventive care.[11]

In Kaiser Permanente's early years, neither prepaid medicine nor group practice was popular or established. As of 1946, some 56 of 368 medical groups with three or more doctors offered prepayment plans of some kind, but these plans generally represented only part of their practice.[12]

While in 1946 the American Medical Association [AMA] never attacked group practice outright, it was always eager to point to its disadvantages, especially the fact that group practice invariably put physicians into an employer-employee relationship ... The medical establishment was also deeply suspicious of the corporate aspects of group practice ... Large medical societies were ... suspicious ... of any form of group medical practice in their area ... Prepayment constituted a threat to the integrity of the physician-patient relationship.[13]

Kaiser Permanente had several factors that inhibited its enrollment besides organized opposition from the AMA. Unions were bound by national bargaining agreements at first and had difficulty working out local options to enroll in Kaiser or other prepaid groups. Also many employers were wary of participating in any medical plan that the AMA disapproved. And typically not all workers in a firm wanted to receive medical care from a group practice plan, and initially employers offered only one type of coverage. Dual choice — so-called because employees were offered Kaiser and one other option — soon became standard practice for groups enrolled in Kaiser.[14]

Dr. Sidney Garfield and Kaiser Permanente were not the first to offer prepaid group plans. As early as 1790, the Boston Dispensary offered group-practice prepaid coverage to its membership. Consolidated Edison Company of New York in 1891 established a prepaid medical care program for its workers. In 1929, the Department of Water and Power of the City of Los Angeles contracted with Drs. Donald Ross and Clifford Loos of the Ross-Loos Medical Group in Los Angeles for prepaid medical coverage for its 12,000 employees and 25,000 dependents.[15]

The first self-consciously radical attempt to reorganize medical care on a prepaid, comprehensive basis came out of the cooperative movement. In 1929, the first medical cooperative in America was formed in rural Oklahoma. During the 1930s and 1940s, a number of others appeared across the country. The medical cooperatives emphasized four principles: group practice, prepayment, preventive medicine and — uniquely — consumer participation. The medical profession was unremittingly hostile. By the end of the decade, its representatives succeeded in convincing most states to pass restrictive laws that effectively barred consumer-controlled plans from operating. The medical cooperatives were unacceptable to the AMA because they subjected physicians' incomes and working conditions to direct control by their clients. The most important new cooperative was organized in Seattle at the end of World War II. By a stroke of fortune, a prepaid clinic in Seattle previously operated on a proprietary basis had just been sold to its physicians. The cooperative was able to buy the clinic in the process of acquiring its own 60-bed hospital, as well as some of the practice the physicians had built up. Unlike many other cooperatives, the Group Health Cooperative of Puget Sound became committed to a policy of expansion, financed by a sale of bonds to its members. Without government assistance, it steadily grew into the largest and most successful cooperative plan in the country. Three decades after it was established, its membership exceeded 200,000 — about a fifth of the Seattle area population.[16]

Recent years have seen the growth of several large medical group practices with significant percentages of their business being prepaid. Southern California has been a breeding ground for many of these groups, including the Friendly Hills HealthCare Network, Mulliken Medical Group, HealthCare Partners, Pacific Physician Services, Bristol Park Medical Group and others. These groups have been pioneers in developing innovative managed care systems and programs.

With the growth of managed care has come greater acceptance of the concept of prepaid contracts, including in the medical community at large. The American Medical Association, once wary of an untried concept, has established policy encouraging a pluralistic system that allows for the development of many types of practice environments, including group practice, capitation and managed care plans. Since 1989, the AMA has had an Office of Group Practice Liaision, designed to address the needs of physicians in groups.

Physician management companies

Another recent development is the growth of physician management companies which provide administrative and operational services and systems to medical groups. These physician management companies, some of which are also known as management services organizations (MSOs), can be for-profit or nonprofit, and can be financed from various capital sources (hospitals, health plans, public and private debt, public and private stock, etc.). Normally, medical groups accessing the services provided by these physician management companies sign long-term service agreements with predetermined fees or fee percentages. In the last few years, several physician management companies have turned to the public equity markets and have raised large sums to assist in financing their affiliations with medical groups. PhyCor Inc., Caremark, Coastal Healthcare and Pacific Physician Services are just a few of the recent startups.

Forms of medical groups

There are two main forms of medical groups: the single-specialty group and the multispecialty group. Single-specialty groups can include only primary care physicians, or only sub-specialists, surgical specialists or hospital-based specialists (e.g., radiologists, anesthesiologists, etc.). Some medical groups are organized as a group practice without walls, which is a collection of solo practices with central services and governance.

Physician organization alternatives[18]

Less integration ◄──────────► More integration						
				Medical groups		
Solo practice	Solo practice: shared lease/staff	PPO	IPA/ PHO	Group practice without walls	Single-specialty group	Multi-specialty group

Integration potential

Structure	Revenues	Expenses	Operations	Culture
Solo practice/PPO	None	None	None	None
IPA/PHO	Partial	None	None	None
Group practice w/o walls	Partial	None	Partial	Partial
Single-specialty group	Full	Full	Full	Full
Multispecialty group	Full	Full	Full	Full

Medical groups are usually legally structured as either professional corporations or partnerships, but several other options are available including medical foundations and limited liability companies (in some states). Medical groups can be nonprofit or for-profit, can have physician and nonphysician owners (if legal under state corporate practice of medicine laws), and can be integrated or nonintegrated with a health system, health plan or other capital partner.

The form of a medical group is sometimes dependent on the surrounding environment. Hospital-based specialists usually are members of single-specialty groups. They contract with the hospitals to which they provide services. Medical schools and teaching hospitals normally have affiliations with faculty multispecialty medical groups. In this era of managed care, many primary care physicians have recently joined primary care groups which are aligned or integrated with health systems, health plans and others. Single-specialty groups of sub-specialists, surgical specialists and hospital-based specialists are usually clustered around one or more of the hospitals they practice in. Other physicians are members of multispecialty medical groups that are freestanding, aligned or integrated with health systems, health plans or others. As noted earlier, some multispecialty groups have developed in rural areas which lack large hospitals and related ancillary services. Various industries, labor unions and other organizations have developed and financed primary care and multispecialty groups to care for their workers and members.

1993 distribution of group practices by size[19]

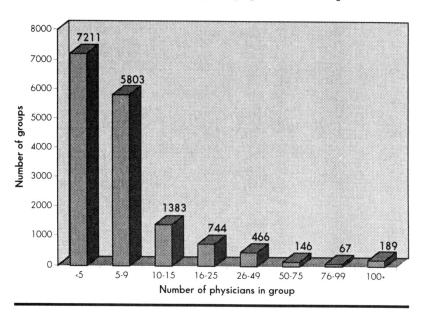

Notes

[1] *Medical Groups in the U.S.*, 1993 Edition, American Medical Association, Chicago, Ill., p. 1.

[2] *The Physician Group Practice*, E. Jordan, p. 1.

[3] Ibid., pp. 15-16.

[4] Ibid., pp. 16-17.

[5] *The Story of the Permanente Medical Group*, John G. Smille, MD, p. 12.

[6] *The Social Transformation of American Medicine*, Paul Starr, 1982, pp. 210-211.

[7] Ibid., pp. 211-212.

[8] *The Physician Group Practice*, E. Jordan, p. 18.

[9] *The Social Transformation of American Medicine*, Paul Starr, 1982, p. 212.

[10] *The Story of the Permanente Medical Group*, John G. Smille, MD, p. 3.

[11] *The Social Transformation of American Medicine*, Paul Starr, 1982, pp. 321-323.

[12] Ibid., pp. 320-321.

[13] *The Story of the Permanente Medical Group*, John G. Smille, MD, pp. 13-14.

[14] Ibid., p. 323.

[15] *The Story of the Permanente Medical Group*, John G. Smille, MD, pp. 10-11.

[16] *The Social Transformation of American Medicine*, Paul Starr, 1982, pp. 302-305, 321.

[17] BDC Advisors Healthcare Consulting Firm, San Francisco, Calif.

[18] *Medical Groups in the U.S.*, 1993 Edition, American Medical Association, Chicago, Illinois, p. 7.

CHAPTER TWO

Forces Driving Physicians to Medical Groups

Growth of managed care

The strongest force driving physicians to join medical groups has been the recent growth of managed care (limited patient choice of physicians and tight cost controls over medical care). In recent years, the growth in managed care has been explosive. Almost two-thirds of the people insured through medium and large companies in 1994 received their care through some kind of managed care arrangement. Medical groups assist physicians in maintaining and enhancing their access to patients who are enrolling in managed care plans. They provide an organized environment that can control health care costs and utilization, as well as demonstrate high quality outcomes.

Recent increase in managed care and decrease in traditional insurance[1]

(large and medium sized companies)

1991   1994

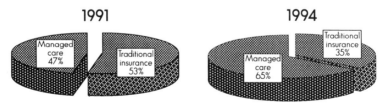

American physicians have experienced dramatic growth of managed care in their practices. In 1994, "at least three-fourths of all doctors signed contracts, covering at least some of their patients, to cut their fees and accept oversight of their medical decisions."[2] Medical groups also have recently increased their percentage of managed care. "Nearly nine out of every 10 medical groups had a contract with an HMO or PPO in 1994. Managed care revenues accounted for 20 percent of total revenues of medical group practices in 1993, up from 17 percent in 1992." [3]

Group practices with managed care contracts[4]

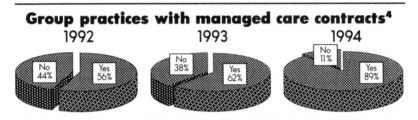

The shift to managed care has been driven by the desire of health care purchasers to reduce their health care costs, which have been increasing exponentially.

Health care spending[5]
(in billions of dollars)

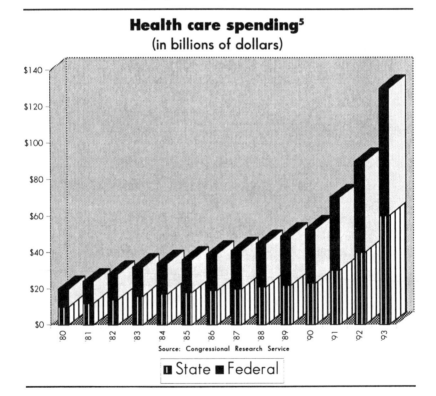

Source: Congressional Research Service

Impact of rising health care costs[6]

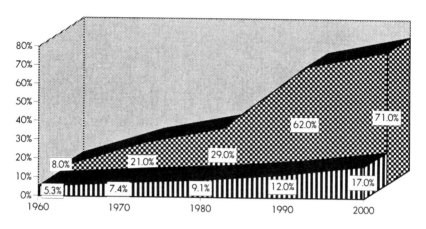

80%
70%
60%
50%
40% — 62.0% — 71.0%
30%
20% — 8.0% — 21.0% — 29.0%
10%
0% — 5.3% — 7.4% — 9.1% — 12.0% — 17.0%
1960   1970   1980   1990   2000

▥ Percentage of GNP ▨ Business spending % of pretax profits

In response to health care purchasers' demands for low-cost health care, health maintenance organizations (HMOs) have offered reduced, all-inclusive prices for their managed care products. They are confident they can manage the costs of health care while still offering good care and making a profit. These HMOs point to examples of cost savings possible under managed care: "In ... California now, the going rate paid by HMOs for heart bypass surgery is $15,000, including all doctors, hospitals and other fees. In contrast, total fees for bypass surgery under traditional insurance in much of the country can easily be $45,000 or more. There is no evidence of any differences in medical outcomes ... Three-fourths of all privately insured patients [in California] are now in HMOs, and even one in four elderly Medicare patients has joined ... In the most recent sign of savings, large employers in the state, in negotiations with fiercely competing HMOs, have obtained rollbacks in health premiums for next year of up to 10 percent." [7]

Fueled by lower HMO premiums, HMO enrollment has grown rapidly in the last few years. Much of the recent growth in HMO enrollment has occurred in markets long immune to HMOs. "The numbers are climbing fast everywhere except in sparsely populated regions." [8]

Reduced hospital days with HMOs[9]

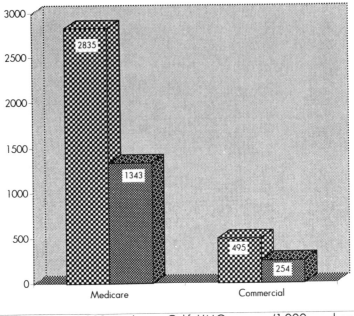

Hospital reimbursement methods used by HMOs[10]

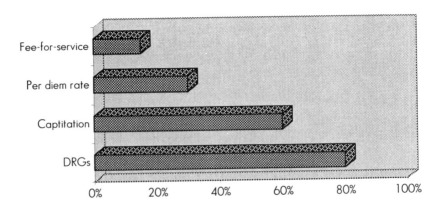

Actual growth of U.S. HMO enrollment, 1984-1994 [11]
(in millions of enrolled lives)

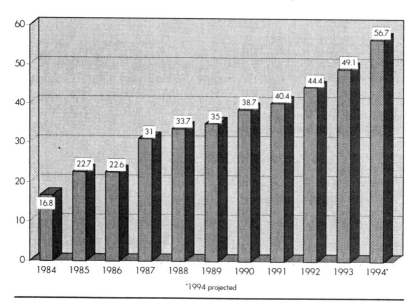

*1994 projected

Health care as big business

Another force driving physicians to medical groups has been the evolution of health care from a cottage industry into the domain of big business that now accounts for one-seventh of the American economy. Health care has become the new "darling" of Wall Street: "Mergers and acquisitions of hospitals; physician groups with their patient lists; medical laboratories; and other patient care services have totaled $20 billion [in 1994]; up from just $6 billion in 1992. Combined with the $22 billion in pharmaceutical deals, health care mergers surpassed in value those of any other industry for 1994."[12] "In just two years one private hospital company, Columbia/HCA Healthcare, has grown from a small regional chain into the owner, when recent deals are completed, of 311 hospitals — half of all the for-profit hospital capacity in the country ... Over the last two years in Southern California, seven large medical systems have gained control over 75 percent of the private insurance market of some 7.2 million people."[13] Many physicians are concerned that if they do not join a large health care organization, they will be left out in the cold.

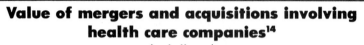

Value of mergers and acquisitions involving health care companies[14]
(in billions)

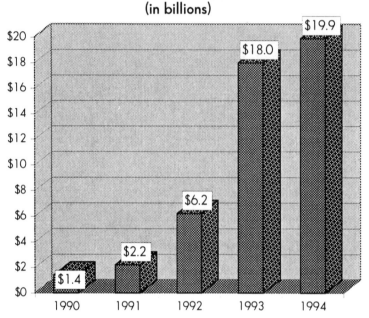

Domestic and non-pharmaceutical companies only

Changed health care environment

In the old health care environment (the fee-for-service system), physicians provided services for patients who either paid the bill themselves or billed the physician charges to their insurance company or the government. As long as the bill was not too high, the patient, insurance company, or government generally paid. Since there was little actual control over health care costs, each year physicians, health systems and insurance companies raised their premiums to the main purchasers of health care: employers and the government.

Under the new health care environment (the managed care system), these traditional health care purchasers have demanded an end to spiraling premium prices. They (and the insurance companies and HMOs) have shifted the risk of controlling health care costs to the providers of care (physicians and health systems). Under this "managed care" system, providers not only accept risk, but are accountable for managing the entire continuum of care for an enrolled patient population. The need for an organized approach to "managing care" has increasingly driven physicians to medical groups. Insurance companies and HMOs generally shift risk to providers in two ways: "discounted fees" and "capitation" (providers receive a set fee per-enrollee per-month).

Changed health care environment

"Old" health care environment	"New" health care environment
• cottage industry; • solo or small physician practices; • physician, patient relationships; • self-directed, patient choice; • diffuse, unintegrated systems; • unmanaged fee-for-service care; • fee increases to cover costs; • multitude of health plan payers; • proliferating, expensive high-tech; and • assumed, unaccountable quality.	• big business; • large medical groups; • physician, health plan relationships; • employer, health plan choice; • broad-based, integrated systems; • managed capitated care; • reduced fees, global budgets; • consolidation of health plan payers; • regional, cost-effective, high-tech; and • accountability for quality, outcomes.

Shift to outpatient and physician care

Another recent major trend affecting the increase in managed care is the shift of hospital business from inpatient care to outpatient care (and physician and medical group care).

A greater percentage of the premium dollar is also moving outside the traditional hospital environment to physician and professional services. This will continue as capitation increases.

The mix of hospital business is changing[15]
from inpatient...

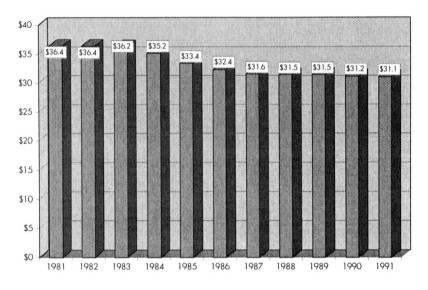

to outpatient

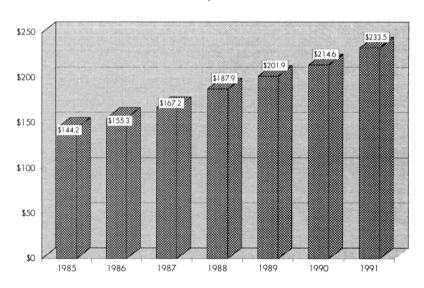

The premium dollar has moved outside the hospital ... to physician services[16]

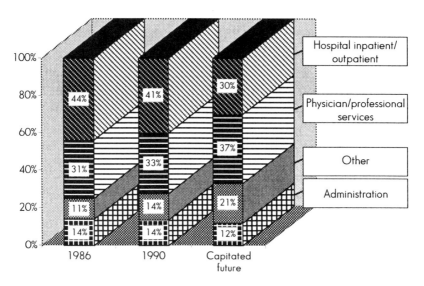

Legend:
- Hospital inpatient/outpatient
- Physician/professional services
- Other
- Administration

Data shown (bottom to top per year):

1986: 14%, 11%, 31%, 44%
1990: 14%, 14%, 33%, 41%
Capitated future: 12%, 21%, 37%, 30%

Changed incentives under capitation

From "managing sickness"	To "managing health"
• episodic care; • optimum individual performance; • hospital-/specialist-focused; • health plan risk management; • paid more for "sickness"; • "Do more, get more"; and • quality care equals extensive care.	• accountable for community health; • optimum health system performance; • primary care/preventive care focused; • provider and self risk management; • paid more for "wellness"; • "Do more, get less"; and • quality care equals effective care.

Old incentives[17]

Hospitals	Physicians
• maximize reimbursement; • increase admissions; • fill beds; and • maximize fee-for-service business.	• maximize "up-coding"; • only take fee-for-service; • maximize number of tests; • stake future on solo practice; and • under-rate primary care.

Changed incentives under capitation

Capitation fundamentally changes the incentives for providers of health care. Under capitation, the amount of reimbursement to providers from health plans is fixed, so more care only results in more provider expenses, which can use up the fixed reimbursements these providers receive. By "managing health" instead of "managing sickness" (easier to do in an organized medical group setting), these providers can keep their expenses low and maximize their profits under capitation.

What about quality?

One of the main concerns about the incentives under capitation is whether quality will suffer when providers receive a preset fee to meet all medical needs. Many physicians are concerned about this "disincentive" for providing care. They claim that lower quality is sure to result (others argue the opposite view). Dr. William S. Andereck, an internist at California Pacific Medical Center in San Francisco, describes why he resigned from an HMO because he felt the incentives were unethical:

> "You get the same amount whether you see the patient or not. For the black and white stuff, they still make the same calls. But most of medicine isn't black and white. It's judgment calls, and that's where the incentive system has its impact. If a woman has a lump in her breast, the doctor can wait three weeks or send her to the surgeon down the hall for an immediate biopsy. Probably the outcome will be the same ... what if it was your wife?"[18]

HMOs and medical groups that have significant capitation experience argue that since they take financial responsibility for a patient's care over time, they actually have an economic imperative to perform useful tests and surgery. These HMOs and medical groups indicate that operating under a capitation system can actually mean better patient care. The emphasis on keeping a patient "well" may contribute to patients living healthier, longer lives with less acute care intervention.

> "The lesson we've learned, and it cost us quite a bit to learn it, is that you do well only by keeping patients well," said John McDonald of the Mulliken group. He noted that poor management of hypertension, diabetes or congestive heart failure can lead to catastrophic expenses. "These delayed procedures this year will cost you far more next year," McDonald said.
>
> In some cases, the detailed scrutiny of medical decisions ... can mean better care for less. The Kaiser plan in southern California, for example, found that by offering Pap smears to women on a scientifically based schedule, in most cases every three years, they could perform fewer total tests on more women. They spent less money, but detected more cases of early cervical cancer ...
>
> HMOs ... reward doctors not only for holding down referrals and tests, but also for improving the rate at which children are immunized and for their scores in privately conducted surveys of consumer satisfaction. They also foster the use of scientific guidelines for care and peer review of doctor's decisions.
>
> "The part of the system that has the best quality, the part of the system that is the most accountable, the part that is best able to present information to the public is the managed care part of the business," said William Roper, former head of the Federal Medicare and Medicaid programs, who is now chief medical officer of Prudential Health Care.[19]

Another common concern is that the lower reimbursements being paid by HMOs to health care providers will result in a lower quality of care. Although this is a very controversial subject, only a few studies of the correlation between the cost of care and the quality of care have been conducted. Part of the difficulty in evaluating quality of care is the current lack of good outcome data. A recent study of 2,024 Medicaid patients by researchers at the Johns Hopkins School of Public Health provides new support for the idea that strategies to contain health care costs do not automatically compromise quality of care.

> Researchers at Johns Hopkins School of Public Health in Baltimore found no evidence that patients treated by low-cost providers for a variety of common conditions got lower quality care as a result ...

"This study supports the premise that providers can do better at containing costs without harming quality," said Neil R. Powe, associate professor of health policy and management at Johns Hopkins ...

Cost-cutting efforts, especially those used by managed care plans, have provoked fierce debate among physicians, policy makers and patients over their impact on patient care. Only a handful of studies have been published that look at the issue with mixed results. In their study, the researchers analyzed ... data and individual charts kept by ... 106 physician practices, 19 hospital outpatient clinics and 10 community health centers ...

Quality indicators included access to care, technical quality and appropriateness of care. The researchers also rated providers in the quality of their medical charts and on how often the patients were hospitalized ...

While researchers found variation in quality, in general, the performance of providers was consistent across cost levels.[20]

Medical group managed care tools

Physicians in medical groups are organized to both manage costs and quality and demonstrate accountability for managed care enrollees better than solo physicians. In addition to having an environment that supports peer review and coordinated cost control, medical groups are structured so that sophisticated tools can be used to manage both quality and utilization of care for "capitated" managed care enrollees.

Solo practitioners have difficulty developing similar tools to manage their capitated managed care enrollees due to lack of integration of their practices as well as limited capital. These solo practitioners usually are dependent on sharing resources with other physicians through agreements with an IPA or PHO. IPAs and PHOs

Managed care tools

Utilization management tools	Clinical care tools
• referral authorizations; • selective provider panels; • prospective/concurrent/retroactive review; • precertification; and • case management.	• critical pathways; • clinical protocols; • managed care information systems; • operational cost control systems; • outcome measurement systems; and • risk management systems.

Case management is a systematic approach to:[21]

- identifying high-risk, high-cost patients;
- accessing opportunities to coordinate care;
- accessing and choosing treatment options;
- developing treatment plans to improve quality and efficacy;
- controlling costs; and
- managing a patient's total care to ensure optimum performance.

frequently have difficulty developing these tools because of the reluctance of their physician and health system members to contribute significant capital. IPAs and PHOs may also have difficulty governing and managing non-integrated physicians. Medical groups can pool resources to develop systems and support services to help manage health care costs. Those medical groups that are integrated with a capital partner such as a health system can develop even more comprehensive managed care tools. Those medical groups that effectively use these tools have a tremendous advantage in attracting managed care contracts over those who do not.

Medical group managed care performance

In a major medical outcomes study commissioned by the Rand Corporation, Santa Monica, Calif., multispecialty medical groups significantly outperformed solo physicians and single-specialty groups in managing costs and utilization. The Rand study analyzed medical outcomes for 20,000 patients, cared for by 349 physicians in three major United States cities with the data adjusted for patient mix.

Study of utilization by medical groups and solo physicians[22]

Ratios	Multispecialty groups	Solo M.D.s & single-specialty groups	% variance
% hospitalized	4.24%	6.94%	+64%
Visits/patient/yr.	4.73	4.30	-9%
Drugs/patient	1.45	1.53	+6%
$ pts. w/tests/visit	38.4%	47.0%	+22%
Mean $ tests/visit	$22.40	$27.40	+22%
Mean $ tests/pt./yr.	$103.70	$113.80	+10%

Please note that the utilization numbers presented for multispecialty group practices represent levels under prepaid delivery; the numbers for solo physicians and single-specialty groups represent fee-for-service delivery.

Deteriorating practice economics

Another major force driving physicians to join medical groups is their deteriorating practice economics, particularly those physicians in solo or small practices.

Physicians have recently seen dramatic decreases in their revenue reimbursements and increases in their costs. According to Cejka & Co., a St. Louis consulting firm, physicians' costs have risen by nearly 50 percent over the five years ended in 1993.[23]

Factors contributing to deteriorating practice economics

- discounting and nominal price increases by payers;
- Medicare and Medicaid discounting and fee reallocations;
- competitive pricing of capitation and other managed care reimbursements to physicians;
- increasing practice overhead and liability costs;
- administrative burdens and paperwork complexity;
- practice restrictions and increased regulations;
- increasing patient loads and patient demands;
- shifting referral patterns between physicians; and
- new practice management requirements – information systems and utilization management.

Declining rate of premium increases

Another factor which has contributed to deteriorating physician practice economics is the recent smaller premium rate increases which have been assessed by insurance companies and HMOs to health care purchasers for conventional, HMO and PPO coverage. These smaller rate increases have contributed to reduced rate increases in reimbursements to providers, as have the large and increased retentions of premium dollars by insurance companies and HMOs to finance their growth and enhance shareholder value: "[In 1993], liquid assets at many HMOs climbed 15 percent or more. Four of the industry's biggest companies each have tucked away more than $1 billion."[28]

Percentage change in physician net income vs. Inflation[25]
1987-1991

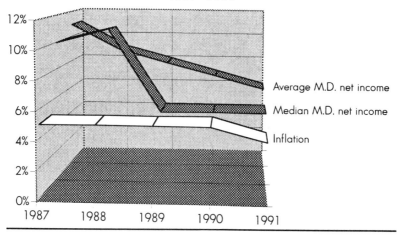

Average M.D. net income

Median M.D. net income

Inflation

Specialist visits decline under managed care[26] [27]

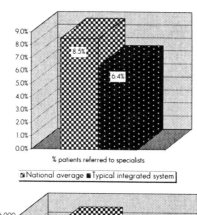

% patients referred to specialists

National average ■ Typical integrated system

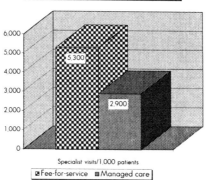

Specialist visits/1,000 patients

Fee-for-service ■ Managed care

Percentage increases (decreases) in health premiums[29]
1991 to 1995

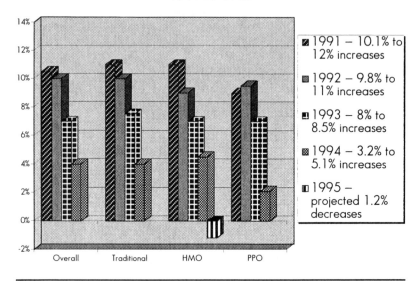

- ▨ 1991 – 10.1% to 12% increases
- ▥ 1992 – 9.8% to 11% increases
- ▣ 1993 – 8% to 8.5% increases
- ▩ 1994 – 3.2% to 5.1% increases
- ▥ 1995 – projected 1.2% decreases

(Categories: Overall, Traditional, HMO, PPO)

Physician quotes[24]

"Our practice is very busy, but administrative and overhead costs coupled with fee discounting make it difficult to prosper as we used to."
— *Active three-physician group*

"If our overhead goes up any more, we will strongly consider leaving private practice and joining Kaiser. We just can't make it ..."
— *A busy four-physician group*

"We are considering scaling down, or possibly adding physician extenders, in order to stay in practice ..."
— *A six-physician group*

"I've been in practice over 10 years and last year only earned $85,000 from the practice. Our (net) revenues are going down, and our overhead is going up. Is it any wonder some physicians ... join Kaiser for $110,000 per year? ..."
— *A "successful" internist*

The need for capital

In the fee-for-service world, capital was not essential for physician and medical group success. Physicians and medical groups would determine projected cost increases, then raise fees to cover these extra costs and keep physician distributable income growing. Equipment and facilities were usually leased in order to minimize cash required for down payments. Systems were kept simple to avoid setting aside any current physician income.

In the managed care and capitated world, capital is becoming essential for physicians and medical groups to succeed. Physicians and medical groups now need sophisticated managed care, information and operational systems to demonstrate accountability for managed care enrollees. Physicians and medical groups also need capital for growing physician networks, demonstrating state-of-the-art technology, quality and service, and absorption and management of risk. Medical groups can provide physicians with organized structures to develop accountable systems and to attract and build capital. However, only a select few medical groups have been successful in capital accumulation. Coddington, Moore and Fischer, of BBC Research and Consulting in Denver, Colo., indicate why most medical groups lack adequate capital:

> The basic financial principles that apply to any business, small or large alike, are also relevant to medical groups, especially primary care practices. A business has to have capital, or access to it, in order to stabilize its operations, including salaries for key

Why do physicians & medical groups need capital?

- To provide and grow competitive, comprehensive physician networks that attract, retain and effectively support and manage payer contracts for broad geographic areas;
- To absorb start-up losses and physician recruitment costs during growth periods;
- To demonstrate state-of-the-art technology, quality and service;
- To develop systems to appropriately measure and demonstrate appropriate outcomes;
- To develop efficient and effective management systems (computerized medical records, management information systems, telecommunication systems, etc.);
- To develop additional sources of revenue and margins over the continuum of care;
- To absorb and manage risk under "capitated" managed care; and
- To keep up with well-capitalized competitors.

professionals, to invest in system improvements and to expand. Given declining net incomes for many physicians in this group, their ability to borrow from normal business sources, such as commercial banks, is limited ... Further, since most medical groups operate on a cash flow basis, they lack funds to invest in building primary care networks.[30]

As managed care payers demand more primary care physicians (and fewer specialists), medical groups are faced with large recruitment and start-up costs for establishing new primary care practices. Coddington, Moore and Fischer estimate the bill facing those developing primary care networks:

> As a rule of thumb, we believe that each primary care practice established in quality facilities in a metropolitan area requires a $200,000 investment per physician spread over the first two or three years. This covers facilities, equipment and initial shortfalls in revenues. In California, it is estimated that this amount approaches $300,000. In rural areas it may be less.
>
> As a general rule, hospitals and health care organizations [and medical groups] seeking to expand their primary care base can expect to pay $50,000 to $75,000 for the first year a new doctor is in practice. This covers recruiting, moving and compensating existing partners in the practice for the loss of income from dilution in the patient base.[31]

Key physician (and medical group) managed care and operational systems

Managed care systems	Operational systems
• claims processing;	• financial reporting;
• member eligibility tracking;	• billing and collecting;
• member services;	• clinical pathways and protocols;
• managed care information services;	• appointment scheduling;
• contract management;	• medical records and transcription;
• utilization management & review;	• materials and facilities management;
• quality assurance, outcome data; and	• human resources; and
• health promotion, preventive care.	• ambulatory services management.

Mean funding — physician organizations[33]

Types of physician organizations	Mean funding requirements (in millions)
• Independent practice associations (IPAs)	$1.2
• Physician/Hospital Organizations (PHOs)	$2.2
• Staff models	$7.8
• Management services organizations (MSOs)	$9.6
• "Freestanding" medical groups	$19.7
• Medical foundations	$20.0

The development of information systems for managed care can also be very costly:

> The amounts being invested in information systems are truly astounding ... from $3 million to $8 million per year [per health care organization] over the next few years ... As one individual said ... "What we have isn't good enough for the future, especially when we are at risk. We simply have to invest now to prepare for the future or we won't be competitive in the marketplace."[32]
>
> Paul Teslow, former CEO of UniHealth [in Southern California], said, "I can't say enough about the importance of information systems ... We have spent $50 million on information systems over the past few years" ... A UniHealth staff member noted that information systems in a capitated system need to provide real-time information so operational changes and decisions can be made quickly. He said that it is important to be able to constantly compare actual utilization against that projected ...
>
> A UniHealth financial manager talked in terms of the need to build an "electronic data interchange." This type of system would include the ability to process claims, prepare reports on patient encounters, determine patient eligibility (e.g., which individuals are eligible for which services, co-payments and deductibles) and a unified medical record. "In addition we want to integrate the records — medical and business — for physicians and hospitals."[34]

Affiliating with a capital partner

Because of the above capital needs, some physicians (and medical groups) are affiliating with capital partners. One medical group, the Fargo Clinic, Fargo, N.D., had several reasons for a hospital affiliation:

Reasons for one medical group affiliating with a hospital[35]

- A preference to join hands with its neighbor and supporter (hospital);
- A hope of achieving economies of scale through less duplication ... The clinic and hospital identified 20 areas for consolidation, including human resources, security, plant maintenance and information systems;
- An ability to position the organization for capitation, including the ability to sign "single signature contracts" covering both the physician and hospital services;
- The need for the clinic to gain access to capital; and
- A desire to do what is best for the people in the service area.

Pros and cons of physicians and medical groups affiliating with a capital partner

Alternative	Pros	Cons
No affiliation	• groups (physicians) maintain independence, control over destiny; • no strings attached; and • flexibility, some leverage with hospitals, HMOs.	• limited capital to grow and compete; • non-integrated health care delivery system; and • well-capitalized competitors.
Affiliation	• adequate capital to grow and compete; • groups (physicians) obtain financial stability; • potential integrated health care delivery system; • sophisticated managed care/operational systems; • enhanced contracting; and • outside expertise.	• high returns to the capital partner; • cultural differences — medical groups (physicians) and the capital partner; • loss of physician autonomy; and • trust, equity and control issues.

Physician (and medical group) sources of capital

Sources of capital	Considerations
• Hospitals and health systems • Health plans	• Allows integration of services and potential lower capital cost • Usually only available in "staff models" – physicians who become health plan employees
• Private and public capital • Traditional debt financing • Physician-generated capital	• Non-integrated financing – usually requires high return to nonphysician investors • Non-integrated financing – usually high debt cost with physician personal guarantees • Physicians usually unwilling to set aside sufficient capital

Physicians and medical groups should first determine their shared visions, goals, objectives and values, then search for a capital partner that is compatible. Physicians and medical groups should proceed carefully, weighing the pros and cons of various affiliation options.

Some physicians and medical groups prefer to stay independent because of the strings attached to a capital partner relationship. The problem with physician and medical group independence is that health plans and health systems (as well as others) can use their significant capital resources to recruit other physicians, to offer a better product to health care purchasers, to absorb managed care risks, and to fund future growth strategies. Though medical group affiliations are underway nationwide, relatively few medical groups have completed affiliations with capital partners.

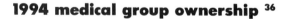

1994 medical group ownership [36]

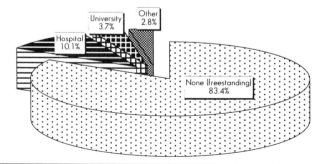

University 3.7%

Other 2.8%

Hospital 10.1%

None (freestanding) 83.4%

1993 medical group affiliations with hospitals[37]

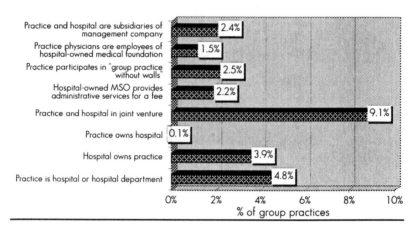

% of group practices

How to upset medical group physicians[38]
Actual quotes from one hospital's correspondence regarding a potential affiliation with a medical group

"We're not interested in a merger with the medical group. There are fears of independent physicians developing a very hostile reaction."

"We can't offer (the potential affiliated) medical group any more than independents ... The hospital should offer no special consideration to (the potential affiliated) medical group."

"Hospitals are there to provide services (for example, lab, CT, MRI, etc.) — doctors are there to supply patients. Hospitals are disinclined to share hospital resources with physicians."

"The hospital's major goal is gaining operational control over the physician practice component of the (potential affiliated) group including:
- the composition of the medical group (by specialty);
- scheduling and hours of medical group operation;
- all physician recruitment and firing;
- the integration of non-group primary care and sub-specialty physicians with the delivery system;
- approval of the institutional and professional components of managed care contracts; and
- employment, termination, compensation and job description of the group medical director."

Barriers to medical groups affiliating with hospitals

There are several barriers that make medical group affiliations with hospitals (especially nonprofit hospitals) difficult to accomplish. This includes the lack of a common shared vision, legal and regulatory issues, trust and control issues, and cultural differences between the parties. Outside consulting advice is often invaluable in assisting affiliation parties to overcome these barriers.

Barriers to physician and medical group affiliations with nonprofit hospitals

Barriers	Nonprofit hospitals	Physicians/medical groups
• No commonly shared vision	• nonprofit, community focused.	• for-profit, internally focused.
• Legal and regulatory issues	• restriction on physician governance in tax-exempt entities (<21%); and • inurement, fraud and abuse laws.	• desire for at least 50 percent shared governance in affiliation entities; and • Stark I and II laws.
• Trust and control issues	• historical mistrust of physician governance; • control over managed care contract allocations; and • control over physicians.	• historical mistrust of hospital motives; • control over amount of physician compensation; and • control over hospital.
• Cultural differences	• large and bureaucratic; • established and diversified; • long-term perspective; • management-controlled; • hierarchical; and • autocratic.	• small and fraternal; • young and diversifying; • short-term perspective; • physician-controlled; • consensual; and • democratic.

The 'bidding wars' for primary care physician practices

Over the last couple of years one of the major forces driving primary care physicians to medical groups has been the bidding wars for primary care physician practices. A "feeding frenzy" has occurred in some markets as hospitals, health plans and others have rushed to better the offers others have made in order to ensure they "own" a sufficient component of primary care physicians in their market to both attract and retain managed care enrollees or "covered lives." In several cases, solo primary care practices are being purchased without adequate thought on how real efficiencies or group culture will be developed (leaving the buyer with an expensive collection of solo practices that may never be able to effectively perform in a managed care environment). Existing medical group practices with primary care physician components are also major targets of acquisition.

Primary care physicians are either becoming direct employees of these buyers (staff models) or are joining or forming medical groups aligned with or integrated with these buyers. Staff models are very controversial in some markets and may be opposed by physicians, who may be concerned that the buyers' motives for directly employing physicians are to "control" physicians or to keep the physicians from "collective bargaining" as a medical group. Some physicians would like to see the tables turned with "physicians directly employing hospital administrators."

> The CEO of a large hospital that is moving aggressively toward employing primary care physicians said that there were several major stumbling blocks. There is the expectation of physicians about the goodwill value of their practice; this can make such a move financially unfeasible for the hospital. Another problem is development of a compensation model that stimulates productivity, works well under capitation, and provides the kind of base salary attractive to physicians who are considering alternatives, such as being employed by the larger clinics or in a staff or group-model HMO ...
>
> Dr. James Todd, president of the American Medical Association, said that, "One of the big concerns is the number of hospitals literally buying up practices and making physicians hospital employees. We do not think that physicians should be employees of hospitals. They should be partners with hospitals."
>
> The direct employment of physicians by a hospital has several drawbacks. Direct hospital employment of physicians can reduce incentives for productivity and typically does not encour-

age the same degree of risk-sharing as other models; thus, it leads to a less effective alignment of financial incentives. It often skews the balance of power to the hospital rather than toward physicians, and in the long run this can lead to less innovation.[39]

The Governance Committee of the Advisory Board Company indicates that the "only downside reported by leading staff-model providers is potential diminution of physician productivity and commitment after onset of the 'nine-to-five' lifestyle. [In addition], the staff model may lack the entrepreneurial spirit desired by some physicians."[40] The Advisory Board Company goes on to state that while physicians employed directly by hospitals usually have straight salary arrangements, there is no reason these physicians cannot be compensated in the same manner as physicians who are not directly employed by hospitals (e.g., with productivity formulas, risk-sharing arrangements that align hospital and physician incentives, capitation compensation formulas, etc.): "Assuming that proper incentives are in place, [there is] no reason to believe that [the] staff model should experience low productivity or compromised quality ... In fact, [the] best systems ensure strong performance through bonus schemes (worth up to 20 percent of base salary) that reward physicians for quality, efficiency and productivity as well as participation in CQI/TQM initiatives." [41]

Direct employment of physicians by hospitals can also result in "full integration" of physicians and hospitals. This contrasts with the "partial integration" achieved through other affiliation methods (MSOs, PHOs, foundations, etc.) as well as other benefits, as outlined by the Advisory Board Company below:

- The staff model is very attractive to primary care physicians because it addresses a number of their pivotal concerns — income, lifestyle and administrative burdens;
- The greatest of these concerns is income security — a key short-term benefit of the staff model is the ability to pay doctors more than they would earn in a non-integrated system;
- Employing physicians is one of the few "safe harbors" under the Internal Revenue Service regulations. While hospitals face legal repercussions from offering practice development assistance or direct income subsidies to independent physicians, employed physicians can be given such assistance;
- The staff model enjoys a major "edge" vis-à-vis contractual models in its ability to attract and retain primary care phy-

sicians, as employment permits direct investment in primary care salaries and practice development;

- The system directly employing physicians can mandate that physician referrals remain in the network;
- The vertically-integrated staff model is the ultimate destination for most major health systems; this model offers the best means to develop a low cost, stable delivery network;
- Staff model physicians are consistently more cost-efficient than the national norm;
- There are two reasons that the staff model is a more efficient entity: 1) the health system is now free to intervene one-to-one with physicians on issues ranging from utilization to productivity; and 2) the staff model encourages system rather than factional loyalty, increasing the ability to make tough strategic decisions and decreasing the likelihood of defection by splinter groups;
- The biggest advantage of the staff model is a unified governance structure — an organization with one board, one CEO, one bottom line is "liberated" to make the difficult strategic choices that forge a sustainable system;
- Because a unified structure blends together what were once clearly individual groups, the staff model also faces lower risks of major defection; and
- The unified staff model also ends one prime source of contention: Physician-hospital rivalry for outpatient business. Since a single organization owns both the hospital and physician practices, both parties benefit from ambulatory growth.[42]

Primary care physician practice purchases are accelerating for a number of reasons with the major reason being the desire of the buyers to capture covered lives to maintain or increase profits and to cover existing costs:

Rationale for primary care physician practice purchases

- The attractiveness of broad, geographically diverse and high-quality networks of primary care physicians to the purchasers of health care;
- Sharing of margins created by effective management of health care costs over the full continuum of care with the assistance of primary care physician "gatekeepers";
- The realization that it takes additional managed care enrollees and aligned primary care physicians to maintain or exceed current non-managed care revenue streams (for hospitals this usually means greatly expanding "covered lives" in order to maintain existing occupancy levels and fixed cost coverage); and
- The desire of the buyers (hospitals, health plans and others) to control or influence "allocations of the managed care dollar" to keep or enlarge their "piece of the pie."

Number of lives required for 65 percent occupancy[43]
400-bed hospital

Payer	Current mix	Current lives	Future mix	Future lives
Medicare HMO	1%	1,312	3%	6,653
Medicare FFS	12%	15,750	12%	26,610
Commercial HMO	43%	56,439	60%	133,050
Commercial FFS	44%	57,752	25%	55,437
Total	100%	131,253	100%	221,750

Historic United States occupancy rates[44]

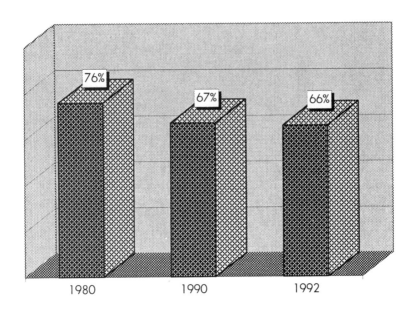

Occupancy in the era of capitation[45]

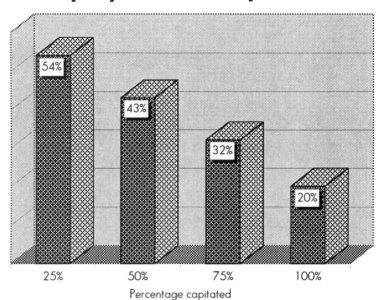

Premium allocations[46]
Traditional insurance vs. HMOs

Premium allocations	Traditional insurance	HMOs	Change
Total premium	$100	$80	(20%)
Delivery system total	$85	$64	(25%)
Primary care physicians	$10	$13	30%
Specialists	$30	$19	(37%)
Hospital	$37	$24	(35%)
Drugs & other	$8	$8	0%
Payer total	$15	$16	7%
Risk management	$6	$5	(17%)
Administration	$5	$5	0%
Profit	$4	$6	50%

Notes
[1] KPMG Peat Marwick, 1994, from "While Congress Remains Silent, Healthcare Transforms Itself," *The New York Times*, Dec. 18, 1994.
[2] "While Congress Remains Silent, Health Care Transforms Itself," *The New York Times*, Dec. 18, 1994.
[3] Marion Merrell Dow, *Managed Care Digest*, Medical Group Practice Edition, 1994, p. 21.
[4] Ibid, p. 23.
[5] "Clinton Considers Stopping Medicaid Under Health Plan," *The New York Times*, March 28, 1994.
[6] "Can Health Insurance Survive," *Integrated Healthcare Report*, October 1993.
[7] "While Congress Remains Silent, Health Care Transforms Itself," *The New York Times*, Dec. 18, 1994.
[8] "While Congress Remains Silent, Health Care Transforms Itself," *The New York Times*, Dec. 18, 1994.
[9] "The Grand Alliance — Vertical Integration Strategies for Physicians and Health Systems," The Advisory Board Company, 1993.
[10] "Direct Connection," Editor: Sue Corrington, Ernst & Young, LLP, Washington, D.C., Jan. 13, 1995.
[11] Marion Merrell Dow, *Managed Care Digest*, HMO Edition, 1994, 1993 ...
[12] Securities Data Company, 1994, from "While Congress Remains Silent, Healthcare Transforms Itself," *The New York Times*, Dec. 18, 1994.
[13] "While Congress Remains Silent, Health Care Transforms Itself," *The New York Times*, Dec. 18, 1994.
[14] Ibid, p. 22 1994 Data through December.
[15] *AHA Hospital Statistics*, 1992-93 Edition, American Hospital Association, Chicago, Ill.
[16] *Source Book of Health Insurance Data — 1992*, Stanford University Hospital; J.P. Morgan; Health Insurance Association of America.

[17] "New Mexico Clinics Without Walls,"*Integrated Healthcare Report*, Editor: John D. Cochrane, M.H.A., February 1993, Los Angeles, Calif., p. 13.

[18] "While Congress Remains Silent, Health Care Transforms Itself," The New York Times, Dec. 18, 1994.

[19] Ibid, p. 22.

[20] Study of Medicaid Patients Concludes Lower Costs Don't Worsen Quality of Care," *Wall Street Journal*, Dec. 28, 1994.

[21] *Ambulatory Care Management and Practice*, Edited by A. Barnett, M.D., and G. Mayer, RN, EdD, FAAN, p. 364.

[22] "Variations in Resource Utilization Among Medical Specialties and Systems of Care," *JAMA*, March 25, 1992.

[23] "Even Before Clinton Reform, Doctors Say They Feel Pinch of Competition," *Wall Street Journal*, March 19, 1993.

[24] Physician interview by BDC Advisors Healthcare Consulting Firm, San Francisco, Calif., 1993.

[25] Sources: American Medical Association, 1992, and BDC Advisors Healthcare Consulting Firm, San Francisco, Calif.

[26] "The Grand Alliance — Vertical Integration Strategies for Physicians and Health Systems," The Advisory Board Company, 1993.

[27] BDC Advisors Healthcare Consulting Firm, San Francisco, Calif.

[28] "HMOs Pile Up Billions in Cash, Try to Decide What to Do With It," *Wall Street Journal*, Dec. 21, 1994.

[29] Sources: "HMOs Plan Price Cuts Averaging 1.2% Amid Lower Costs, Rising Members," *The Wall Street Journal*, Dec. 18, 1994, and KMPG Peat Marwick, 1994/GHAA, 1994.

[30] Integrated Health Care Reorganizing the Physician, Hospital and Health Plan Relationship," Coddington, Moore and Fischer, 1994, p. 148.

[31] Ibid p. 79.

[32] Ibid, p. 80.

[33] "Capital Survey of Emerging Healthcare Organizations," *Integrated Healthcare Report*, Nov. 1994.

[34] "Integrated Health Care: Reorganizing the Physician, Hospital and Health Plan Relationship," Coddington, Moore and Fischer, 1994, p. 137.

[35] "Integrated Health Care: Reorganizing the Physician, Hosptial and Health Plan Relationship," Coddington, Moore and Fischer, 1994 p. 54.

[36] Medical Group Management Association membership database, January 1, 1995.

[37] Marion Merrell Dow, *Managed Care Digest*, Medical Group Practice Edition, 1994, p. 5.

[38] Correspondence from Memorial Hospital to Gould Medical Group, Inc. (100-physician multispecialty group), Modesto, Calif. 1991-1992.

[39] "Integrated Health Care Reorganizing the Physician, Hospital and Health Plan Relationship," Coddington, Moore and Fischer, 1994, pp. 52-53.

[40] "The Grand Alliance — Vertical Integration Strategies for Physicians and Health Systems," The Advisory Board Company, 1993.

[41] Ibid, p. 352.

[42] Ibid, pp. 319-348.

[43] *HMO Industry Profile*, 1992 Edition, and GHAA; "Source Book of Health Insurance Data — 1992," Health Insurance Association of America.

[44] "Capitation Strategies," Integrated Healthcare Report, Dec. 1994.

[45] Ibid.

[46] "Power Notebook," Nathan Kaufman, *Hospitals and Health Networks*, Feb. 5, 1995, p. 60.

CHAPTER THREE

Benefits of Medical Groups for Physicians

In addition to the previously noted forces driving physicians to join medical groups, various inherent benefits of medical groups help them attract and retain physicians.

A 'sharing' environment

Many physicians are attracted to medical groups because of their sharing environments. Medical group physicians like sharing practices with their colleagues, call coverage with a broader group of physicians and access to a ready source of patients. Combining medical records creates a de facto process of peer review, and close proximity of group physicians allows continuous cross-education. Most medical groups have developed formalized peer review processes: "In 1993-94, 83 percent of all groups had formalized peer review processes, while 51 percent had formalized medical review committees." [1] In addition, having physician peers who can counsel, review and give support provides an environment in group practice that is not possible in solo practice:

> Group practice gives the [opportunity for] the physician to practice his [her] specialty and to do only those procedures for which he [she] is best qualified. It gives the physician an opportunity to improve himself [herself] professionally, continuously by contact with his [her] partners and intermittently by the chance to get away for advanced study ... It makes life easier. By proper scheduling of time off, his [her] patients can be adequately cared for at all times ...
>
> The solo physician often lacks the wholesome stimulation arising from close association with other doctors. The average doctor will sharpen his [her] diagnostic acumen and increase his [her] knowledge and ability if he [she] is working with others. He [she] is obliged to keep abreast of the constant advances in his [her] field. It is difficult to hide errors in a group ... [2]

The benefits of large medical groups

New graduating medical students are joining large medical groups (such as Kaiser Permanente and the Mayo Clinic) because of the various benefits they offer:

Benefits of large medical groups for physicians	

• regionally, vertically and horizontally integrated systems;
• guaranteed competitive base salaries;
• comprehensive benefit packages;
• longevity and merit raises;
• opportunities for partnership;
• educational and vacation time off; and
• security and lifestyle advantages.
	• stable, long-term employment;
	• low physician attrition;
	• no buy in or startup costs; and
	• market attractiveness:
	  - systems to manage risk/quality;
	  - competitive pricing;
	  - geographic access; and
	  - broad physician networks.

Harvey MacKay, a best-selling author, describes how the Mayo Clinic, achieves success:

If the Mayo Clinic were ranked in the Fortune 500 last year [1993] it would have been No. 267 ... Mayo generates over $1.6 billion in revenues and annually sees over 320,000 patients ... from over 150 countries ... They have a reputation as the best in the world and it's one they've rightfully earned.

I checked into Mayo a few weeks ago for a minor tuneup ... I witnessed Nordstrom's service, Pepsi's innovation, General Electric's management and 3M's technology, all rolled into a corporate culture.

Surprisingly, several studies have shown the costs per person at Mayo to be 15 percent to 22 percent below the national average ... This is not "low bid meeting specs" health care. It's world-class quality, delivered by doctors who were awarded the Nobel Prize for pioneering the use of cortisone and who also introduced other innovations, like CT scanning ...

The key is the team approach. Mayo's great strength both in delivering quality health care and in cost containment is its comprehensiveness, its ability to provide one-stop shopping for the diagnosis and treatment of practically any medical problem ... The decisions are based on institutional reputations, not individual ones. And yet at Mayo they make you feel you are their only patient and they really do care about you.

Mayo stands as the preeminent symbol of quality in health care. The elements are: teamwork; quality facilities and equipment; quality personnel on every level, from the most menial position to the highest; obsessive cleanliness; and fanatical attention to detail ...

The patient's needs come first ... Lots of rest rooms. Good lighting. Phones answered promptly. Pleasant, smiling, caring people ...[3]

John G. Smillie, M.D., in his history of Kaiser Permanente, states that a National Advisory Commission reported that:

> The quality of care provided by Kaiser is equivalent, if not superior to, that available in most communities. Permanente physicians use standard medical practices and procedures. Patient satisfaction is indicated by the overall flow of patients into Kaiser ... The majority of savings achieved by Kaiser results primarily from effective control over the nature of medical care that is provided.[4]

In spite of the benefits of large medical groups, in 1995, "72 percent of medical groups had 10 or fewer full-time equivalent physicians."[5]

Higher primary care physician incomes in medical groups

Primary care physicians generally earn more in medical groups than in solo practice. This is because of factors found only in an organized medical group structure including: (i) the sharing of income generated from medical group capitation allocations, ancillary services, midlevel providers, and medical group specialists with medical group primary care physicians; and (ii) the additional income generated from effective practice management, increased physician productivity, efficient clinical operations and contract leverage.

Primary care physician (PCP) compensation[6]
(percent of net revenues, 1992 data)

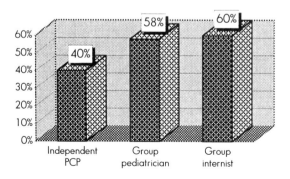

Higher primary care physician annual net incomes in medical groups (1992 data)[7]

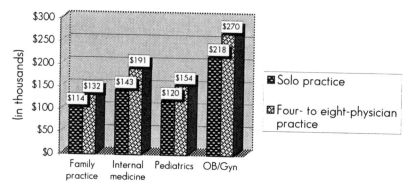

Some sources of increased physician compensation in medical groups

- shared medical group income;
- retention of revenues generated by medical groups;
- reduced physician administrative time – increased physician productivity;
- the benefits of larger size;
- effective practice management;
- improved clinical efficiency;
- use of midlevel providers;
- increased contract leverage with payers;
- shared hospital/specialty services risk-pool bonuses;
- reduced physician risk for group operations; and
- reduced practice startup costs.

Shared medical group income

One of the cornerstones of successful multispecialty medical groups (and primary care groups integrated with health systems) is sharing fee-for-service or capitated income generated by group primary care physicians' internal referrals to group specialists and ancillary services (and integrated health systems) with these primary care physicians through a group compensation plan, profit-sharing plan or capitation allocation plan. Such sharing of income can result in all parties winning in both fee-for-service and capitated environments through higher primary care incomes, stable and profitable referrals to specialists and ancillary services (and integrated health systems), and lower "cost" specialist and ancillary services under capitation. Coddington, Moore and Fischer describe ways to share capital and income with primary care physicians:

> There are basically four ways to generate capital for the expansion of primary care — transfers from the earnings of specialists, income from ancillaries (lab, X-ray, pharmacy), health plan profits or loans or other assistance from hospitals and health plan systems ...
>
> Does this constitute a subsidy of primary care? Some individuals interviewed, usually specialists, often referred to it in these terms ... To focus on primary care subsidies is to "suboptimize" the revenues and profits of the system. One physician said, "You don't hear Kaiser Permanente talking about subsidizing primary care. They think in terms of the whole system, and if the system is working, they could care less about whether or not primary care is being subsidized ..."
>
> We found several cases in which specialists were willing to support primary care physicians even though it meant lower income for themselves. We conclude that one of the secrets of success ... is ... cultures that encourage this kind of sharing. [8]

Retention of revenues generated by medical groups

One major advantage of medical groups is their ability to retain revenues generated by internal referrals for specialist and ancillary services. For fee-for-service business, this means keeping revenues generated from specialist and ancillary services within the medical group. For capitated business, this means keeping margins made on capitated dollars available for these services within the medical group. Several large groups have either developed their own ancillary services or subcontracted for them based on "make or buy" decisions (to capture the margins available from these services on both fee-for-service and capitated business). According to case studies conducted by Coddington, Moore and Fischer, several large groups integrated with hospitals have their ancillary services based at the medical group, not at the hospital:

"Ownership of ancillaries was an interesting issue in nearly all of the case studies. In the Marshfield and Carle Clinic cases, the hospitals generate very little ancillary income; nearly all of it goes to the clinics who own or control radiology, laboratory and pharmacy. The added income contributes to the ability of these clinics to support their primary care networks."[9] For those medical groups choosing to 'make' ancillary services, capital must be generated internally or externally.

"As Jeff Goldsmith, a business consultant, points out, group practices are vertically integrated forms of production with two outputs, physician services and ancillary services such as X-rays and laboratory tests ... large groups may generate substantial profits from ancillary services. 'Ancillary profits,' notes Goldsmith, 'are a significant incentive for the formation of groups, one which is likely to become more powerful as market pressures reduce the profitability of the physician services component of what a practice produces." [10]

Examples of some medical group ancillary services:

- pharmacy;
- laboratory;
- physical therapy;
- occupational therapy;
- cardiac rehabilitation;
- EKGs, EEGs;
- ambulatory surgery;
- optical and audiology;
- MRI and CT;
- radiology and mammography;
- radiation therapy;
- nuclear medicine;
- occupational medicine;
- immediate care;
- gastroenterology lab; and
- home health.

Percentage of all medical groups offering various ancillary services: [11]

Ancillary Services	1994	1993	1992
X-ray (diagnostic and therapeutic)	54.3%	56.0%	57.3%
Clinical laboratory	39.7%	41.3%	42.7%
X-ray (therapeutic)	6.4%	6.4%	6.7%
Immediate care	17.9%	18.3%	18.4%
Physical therapy	16.2%	17.2%	18.3%
Audiology	15.9%	16.8%	18.3%

The use of margins generated by ancillary services by physicians and medical groups providing referrals has been under attack in recent years. Federal legislation (Stark I and II) prohibits physicians and medical groups who provide referrals to ancillary services from financially benefiting from such services. These laws have provided special exemptions for some medical group ancillary services. Some medical groups have formed entities (such as medical foundations) from which physicians do not financially benefit that hold ancillary services.

Another possible source of retained revenues for medical groups are profits or lower administrative costs generated by medical group-aligned or owned health plans. These profits or lower costs can help them grow their primary care networks. Coddington, Moore and Fischer give examples of several medical groups which use health plan profits:

> Profits from health plans were contributing to the cost of expanding the primary care network and to maintaining the incomes of primary care physicians. This was most noteworthy in the cases of Marshfield, Geisinger and Carle Clinics where HMO profits were relatively large. Kaiser Permanente uses the cash flow generated by its health plan to help cover the costs of maintaining its system of primary care offices throughout most of the metropolitan area it serves. [12]

Reduced physician administrative time — increased physician productivity

Using central administration in a group practice to deal with personnel, billing, paperwork, etc., can significantly reduce the time physicians spend doing administrative duties. It allows them to spend more of their time practicing medicine. Abt reports that medical groups spend 4.2 minutes per insurance claim and four hours per week on administrative activities, while solo physicians spend 9.6 minutes per insurance claim and 15 hours per week on administrative activities.[13] Medical group physicians must use their extra time to actually be more productive. (Medical group physicians may be less productive than their solo practice peers because of a different lifestyle.)

Due to economies of scale, the larger the medical group, the smaller the percentage of total staff that is administrative: "[In 1992], administrative staff was 47 percent of nonprovider staff per physician in small group practices, 42 percent to 44 percent of staff per physician in middle-sized groups and 40 percent of staff per physician in large medical groups." [14]

Primary care physicians spend 17 percent of their practice time on administration [15]

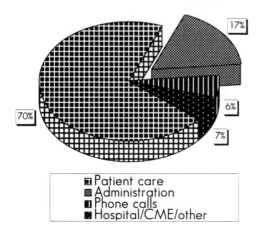

- Patient care
- Administration
- Phone calls
- Hospital/CME/other

Physicians are working harder ...

Average number of hours worked by physicians per week [16]

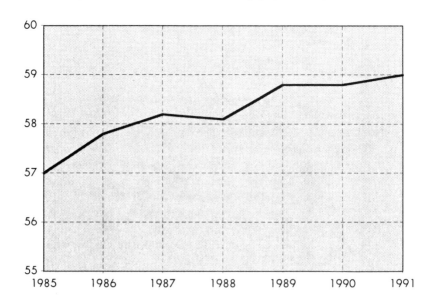

Visits/patient and work/patient [16]

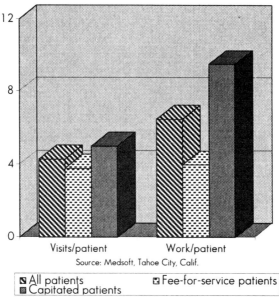

Source: Medsoft, Tahoe City, Calif.

☒ All patients   ☒ Fee-for-service patients
☒ Capitated patients

For less ...

Comparison of fee-for-service and capitated patient dollars/visit and dollars/work unit [18]

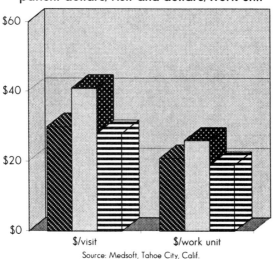

Source: Medsoft, Tahoe City, Calif.

☒ All patients   ☒ Fee-for-service patients
☐ Capitated patients

... with more stress [19]

- 30 percent to 50 percent of doctors would opt against medical school if they had to do it over. At Unum Life Insurance, a major physician insurer, disability claims jumped 60 percent to $1.38 million in the first six months of 1994. Most of the claims involve some impairment.

- Across the country, new programs are emerging to deal with the problem of physician stress. The Center for Physician Development has seen 60 stressed-out physicians (since 1992). The Center for Professional Well-Being counsels some 200 physicians a year. Menninger Clinic counsels some 100 physicians yearly, an increase of about 40 percent in the past 10 years.

Other factors

Medical groups seem to be unable to achieve true economies of scale as they grow larger. The additional layers of bureaucracy, committees and other factors present in many large groups may offset the benefits of size. In addition, according to experts, "economies of scale in physicians' services are limited; the optimal size of a physician group may be only about six physicians." [20] Sometimes, having convenient locations for patients limits available economies of scale: "61.1 percent of medical groups had branch or satellite offices in 1994 ... The average number of branch offices was 3.5 per medical group."[21] Others argue that economies should not be expected as groups grow. Coddington, Moore and Fischer state:

> "Economies of scale by combining solo practice physicians into medical groups are often illusory. Although newly formed, or merged, medical groups are frequently advised that expected financial benefits from improved economies of scale, primarily from spreading overhead over a larger base of patients, probably won't be significant, hope often abounds ... The experts appear to be correct. In our research we saw little evidence of significant economies of scale as the result of combining medical groups into larger practices, or combining groups of physicians with one or more hospitals." [22]

However, there are several areas where medical groups can derive benefits from being larger.

Medical group benefits of larger size

- centralized billing, accounting and other administrative services;
- enhanced systems support (management information services, managed care services, etc.);
- typing and transcription pools;
- efficient space utilization (shared reception, medical records, etc.);
- centralized human resources and recruitment functions;
- personnel pools and temporary staff for vacations;
- savings on medical insurance and other benefits;
- centralized purchasing of supplies, equipment and liability insurance;
- negotiated lower ancillary prices; and
- increased leverage in accessing capital and revenue streams.

Effective practice management

Pooling physician revenues and costs allows physicians in medical groups access to improved practice management services and staff as well as administrative services (both inside and outside). These administrative services, including legal, accounting, consulting, strategic planning and marketing, are usually not affordable by solo physicians. In general, the larger the medical group, the more qualified (and highly compensated) the administrative staff. "Physicians are increasingly in need of more sophisticated management to keep up with the complexities of the health care industry ... Physicians ... are accessing the management capabilities and business systems that medical groups provide." [23]

Medical group practice management benefits

- one highly trained administrator, instead of multiple office managers; and

- access to sophisticated support systems:
  - management information service;
  - managed care systems and services;
  - operational systems;
  - legal, financial, and outside services;
  - marketing and business development; and
  - strategic and financial planning.

Improved clinical efficiency

Shared governance, clinical protocols and shared office space and staff can help physicians better facilitate coordination of clinical care in an efficient manner. As shown on previous page, this can result in better outcomes in a medical group.

Contributors to improved medical group clinical efficiency

- collegial information sharing:
  - physicians updated on new diagnostic techniques;
  - better sharing of ideas and information between physicians and nonphysician staff;
  - consistent utilization review and quality assurance protocols;
  - jointly determined ancillary tests; and
  - shared continuing medical education;
- common quality control programs;
- shared and jointly used equipment and personnel;
- improved backup and call coverage; and
- increased financial capability to purchase state-of-the-art equipment and track outcome data.

Use of midlevel providers

Using midlevel providers (e.g., nurse practitioners and physician assistants) in medical groups allows physicians and medical groups to generate additional compensation and profits by providing care at a lower cost. Physicians who historically were reluctant to hire midlevel providers increasingly turn to them for assistance as managed care increases. An American Group Practice Association focus group composed of physician executives of group practices around the nation predicted in 1994 that midlevel provider use will accelerate in the future:

> Medical groups will make more use of midlevel practitioners in coming years to handle many routine aspects of patient care, such as strep throat and other common illnesses. This will free physicians to spend more time with patients who need more attention and for whom diagnosis and treatment are more complex. Group practices already reengineering their operations to accomplish this goal are finding that doctors like it, patients like it, and physicians are able to interact with patients much more effectively than before. [24]

Under fee-for-service medicine, midlevel providers can be billed out at physician rates and compensated for their services with lower salaries than physicians, creating margins for supervising physicians and medical groups. Under capitated medicine, using midlevel providers instead of expensive physicians saves capitated dollars. As long as midlevel providers are properly supervised by physicians, quality care can be maintained.

More use of midlevel providers in medical groups with managed care (1993 data)

Midlevel compensation/full-time physician [25]

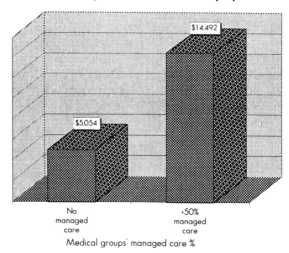

Medical groups' managed care %

Midlevel providers/full-time physician [26]

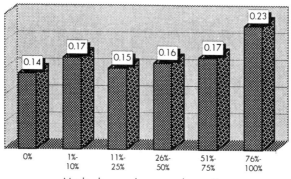

Medical groups' managed care %

Increased contract leverage with payers

Medical groups (especially those groups with large primary care physician components) who have achieved adequate size, geographic coverage and the ability to deliver and manage large blocks of managed care enrollees substantially increase their contract leverage with payers. This usually results in enhanced market share, better rates for physician services, and longer-term managed care contracts. As primary care-oriented physician networks grow larger and become established, they generally increase their percentage of managed care revenues. In 1994, large medical groups had a greater percentage of capitated contract revenues than smaller medical groups: "Multispecialty medical groups with 10 or fewer physicians had 6.2 percent prepaid revenues, medium-sized groups reported between 8.6 percent and 12 percent prepaid revenues, and large multispecialty groups with more than 150 physicians had 28 percent prepaid revenues." [27]

Jan McCormick, Medical Contracts Administrator of CIGNA Corporation, describes the importance of primary care physician networks to health plans:

> From [the health plan] point of view, primary care physician networks tend to be very powerful, thus difficult to negotiate with. Networks can set their own terms. As a result, in trying to penetrate a market, we are forced to accept those terms or negotiate elsewhere. [28]

The health care solar system

Ptolemaic view

Copernican view

PCP = Primary care provider
Source: Bruce Spivey, M.D., president, Northwestern Network

Sharing of hospital/specialty services 'risk-pool' bonuses

Medical groups with capitated managed care contracts can sometimes enhance physician incomes through effective management of hospital and specialty costs, resulting in these groups sharing in year-end risk-pool bonuses with hospitals, specialists and/or health plans. "The difference in unit price between inpatient and outpatient services is especially significant. A hospital day has an average price that exceeds $1,000. The average price of an outpatient encounter is less than $50. The expense of programs to reduce hospitalizations and shorten lengths of stay through precertification, concurrent review, discharge planning, case management and second surgical opinions can be easily offset by relatively small percentage reductions in costly hospital days." [29]

Multispecialty medical groups generally have lower utilization statistics (lower hospital visits and specialty consultations) than single-specialty medical groups:

Number of hospital visits and specialty consultations in medical groups (1994 data) [30]

Specialty	Single-specialty groups	Multi-specialty groups	Percentage difference
Family practice	380	312	+21.8%
Internal medicine	742	679	+9.3%
Pediatrics	318	280	+13.6%
General surgery	489	328	+49.1%

Reduced physician risk for group operations

One benefit some medical groups provide to physicians is reduced risk for how well "the business does." In some medical groups, physicians have no equity at risk, and are only compensated for services rendered. Of course, if physicians have reduced risk for medical group losses, they probably also have a reduced potential for medical group profits (and someone else is taking the risks and rewards).

Reduced risks for physicians in some medical groups

- reduced or eliminated responsibility for overhead;
- stable, long-term employment contracts;
- regular hours, set salaries and benefits;
- set call coverage and vacation;
- comprehensive retirement benefits; and
- enough size, geographic coverage and reserves for long-term security.

Reduced practice startup costs

Formidable economic barriers are discouraging physician graduates from entering solo practice ("buy ins," costs of starting practice, etc.). This is especially true for primary care physicians who may be unable to make sufficient incomes in solo practice to pay off the debts created from establishing a new primary care practice. Most large medical groups have little or no economic barriers for new physicians. Some medical groups even assist new physician recruits in repayment of their medical school loans. Of course, large medical groups also have startup costs, but they can use reserves and ancillary revenues to help fund these capital expenditures. Those medical groups that have eliminated physician "buy ins" and other startup costs have significant advantages in recruiting new physicians.

Other benefits

There are other benefits of medical groups that are not easy to measure. Having someone available to keep a practice going when an unexpected illness or family emergency occurs, working collaboratively with a team of professionals, pride in the quality of care and service provided by the medical group, a steady and diverse patient base, instant feedback on clinical performance, set vacation and continuing medical education time allocations and pay, the security of guaranteed compensation, secure retirement benefits, and an environment to foster social interactions and long-lasting friendships are just some of the benefits for physicians that are only possible in a medical group environment.

Smaller medical group practices are expected to ally themselves with other small groups in confederations so they develop the critical mass and the interdependent-physician culture necessary to successfully deliver coordinated primary and specialty care to defined patient populations. Physicians in small groups and in solo practices can no longer be independent, whether they like it or not. They must learn to work in interdependent teams. [31]

Notes

[1]   Marion Merrell Dow, *Managed Care Digest*, Medical Group Practice Edition, 1994.

[2]   *The Physician Group Practice*, E. Jordan, p. 42.

[3]   "Mayo's Prescription for Success is Something Others Should Copy," Harvey MacKay, United Feature Syndicate, Oct. 23, 1994.

[4]   "The Story of the Permanente Medical Group," John G. Smillie, M.D., p. 219.

[5]   Medical Group Management Association membership database, January 1, 1995.

[6]   1992 Virginia Mason Clinic Survey of Medical Groups.

[7]   "Physician Marketplace Statistics, 1992," American Medical Association, pp. 81-83, 1992.

[8]   "Integrated Health Care: Reorganizing the Physician, Hospital and Health Plan Relationship," Coddington, Moore and Fischer, 1994, p. 148.

[9]   Ibid., p. 84.

[10]   "The Social Transformation of American Medicine," Paul Starr, p. 425.

[11]   Medical Group Management Association membership database, January 1, 1995.

[12]   "Integrated Health Care: Reorganizing the Physician, Hospital and Health Plan Relationship," Coddington, Moore and Fischer, 1994, p. 84.

[13]   "Administrative Costs and the Debate about U.S. Health System Reform: A Review of the Literature," A report by Abt to the Workgroup on Health Care Administrative Costs and Benefits, February, 1993.

[14]   "Integrated Health Care: Reorganizing the Physician, Hospital and Health Plan Relationship," Coddington, Moore and Fischer, 1994, p. 24.

[15]   "Percentage of Practice Time Spent in Various Activities," *The Physician's Advisory*, p. 4., April 1992.

[16]   "Even Before Clinton Reform, Doctors Say They Feel Pinch of Growing Competition," *Wall Street Journal*, March 19, 1993.

[17]   *Physician's Managed Care Report*, January 1995, p. 10.

[18]   Ibid., p. 10.

[19]   What's Up Doc? Stress and Counseling," *Wall Street Journal*, Jan. 10, 1995.

[20]   "The Social Transformation of American Medicine," Paul Starr, 1982, p. 425.

[21]   Medical Group Management Association membership database, January 1, 1995.

[22]   "Integrated Health Care: Reorganizing the Physician, Hospital and Health Plan Relationship," Coddington, Moore and Fischer, 1994, p. 149.

[23]   Ibid., p. 149.

[24]   Ibid., p. 32.

[25]   Ibid., p. 3.

26 "Managed Care Impacts M.D. and Administrator Pay, Use of PAs," *Physician's Marketing and Management*, Dec. 1994.

27 *MGMA Cost Survey: 1995 Report Based on 1994 Data*, 1995, pp. 70, 82.

28 Jan McCormick, Medical Contracts Administrator, CIGNA Corporation, Marion Merrell Dow, *Managed Care Digest*, 1991.

29 *Ambulatory Care Management and Practice*, Edited by A. Barnett, M.D. and G. Mayer, R.N., Ed.D., FAAN, p. 244.

30 *MGMA Physician Compensation and Production Survey: 1995 Report Based on 1994 Data*, 1995, p. 65.

31 *MGMA Physician Compensation and Production Survey: 1995 Report Based on 1994 Data*, 1995, p. 65.

CHAPTER FOUR

Forming a Medical Group

Forming a medical group from scratch is a complicated, costly and challenging endeavor in the new managed health care environment. In the old days, little capital was required to get a medical group up and running. Many groups were founded by a few physicians with little or no startup capital. As physicians, hospitals and others scramble to get medical groups organized for managed care, important steps essential for long-term group success are sometimes missed. The following discussion highlights lessons others have learned the hard way in forming medical groups.

Letters of interest

The first step in developing a new medical group is to get physicians interested in joining. The benefits and challenges of medical groups should be articulated and potential physician leaders identified. Those physicians who are interested in joining a new group should sign a nonbinding letter of interest. This letter affirms their willingness to participate in a group feasibility study, to provide practice profiling information, and to support the efforts of a group formation steering committee.

Establishment of a steering committee

Identifying who will be responsible and accountable for forming the new medical group is the next step in the group formation process. Usually a steering committee is composed of key physician leaders and others who can facilitate group formation.

Group development steering committee

- develop a work plan;
- coordinate formation process:
  - feasibility assessment;
  - business planning;
  - pre-implementation; and
  - implementation;
- communicate with physicians, others;
- broaden physician interest and participation.

- recognized leaders (physician and administrative);
- able to effectively communicate;
- sound financial understanding;
- group-oriented, not self-oriented;
- team players;
- committed to formation process; and
- intelligent, experienced, competent, good listeners.

Development of a group formation work plan

Effective design of a work plan is key to successful formation of a medical group. Work plans should have clearly assigned responsibilities and should be monitored on an ongoing basis. Experience indicates that expected time frames are rarely conservative enough — inevitably what can go wrong will go wrong. Work plans should be dynamic and flexible documents as every market and situation is different. There is no one right way to form a medical group. An example of medical group formation work plan outline follows:

Medical group formation work plan outline

Phase I: Feasibility assessment	Phase II: Business planning	Phase III: Pre-implementation	Phase IV: Implementation
• group vision; • physician selection criteria and mix; • practice profiles; • practice valuations; • market assessment; and • initial financial assessment.	• legal structure; • ownership; • governance; • compensation and work effort; • business plan; and • preliminary legal documents.	• management; • finalize legal documents; • practice merger proposals; • site planning; and • implementation plan.	• office consolidations; • operations; • management information systems; • managed care systems; and • contracting and marketing.

PHASE I: FEASIBILITY ASSESSMENT

Before embarking on formation of a group, it is very important that a feasibility assessment be completed. Development of a shared group vision, determining which physicians will be eligible to participate in the group, practice profiling of the potential physicians joining the group, assessing the market environment and estimating costs of formation and funding sources are essential steps to avoid future problems. Some health systems and physicians have formed medical groups without an adequate feasibility assessment and then found they couldn't pay the bills or had to clean up a big mess.

Group vision and guiding principles

The most important step in forming a successful medical group is establishing a group vision and guiding principles. If the potential group physicians are not willing to follow the group vision and guiding principles, the long-term feasibility of the group is in question. Frequently physicians and hospitals forming groups rush to pick a structural model without first establishing what they are trying to accomplish. It's like buying a computer before finding out if the software you want will run on it first.

The process of developing a group vision and guiding principles establishes a philosophical foundation for the future decision making of the group as well as physician performance parameters. Groups that miss this step may end up without a group culture where physician members just want to look out for themselves. The importance of having a vision explicitly stated and then gaining consensus about the vision is twofold. First, the very act of arriving at an agreement about the vision creates a powerful bond that can sustain a group through the conflicts inherent in the health care industry today. Second, a vision provides a direction, albeit general, that can guide groups through the incredible ambiguity of today's marketplace.[1]

Each group should have its own group vision and guiding principles based on the environment and shared values and objectives. An example of a vision and guiding principles a group might adopt follows:

Sample group vision and guiding principles

The group will:
- deliver high quality, cost-efficient health care;
- offer an attractive, collegial, humanistic, professionally and economically rewarding practice alternative;
- balance the needs of itself and its physician partners;
- consider first, the interests of the patient; second, the interests of the group; and third, the interests of each physician;
- be economically self-sustaining;
- not incur any debt except pursuant to a business plan;
- be committed to developing and supporting managed care and capitated business;
- be focused on serving community health status needs; and
- support education, research and innovation in health care delivery.

Physician selection criteria and mix

Medical groups rise and fall based on the quality of their physicians. Successful groups look for physicians who share their values and understand the need for balancing physician autonomy with group goals and objectives. Developing physician selection criteria that will result in the best physicians joining a group is key.

Sample group physician selection criteria
- professional competence:
  - active membership and good standing on a local hospital medical staff;
  - board certified (or eligible) or postgraduate training acceptable to specific academy;
  - specialty consistent with the needs of the group;
  - professional skill/credentials reviewed, including any disciplinary matters;
  - favorable malpractice sensitivity and record;
  - participant in Continuing Medical Education (CME) and new specialty developments; and
  - good professional judgment and diagnostic ability;
- group relations and participation:
  - shared vision/goals/values of the group;
  - interest in group practice;
  - ability to attract patients/enrollees to the group;
  - ability to understand and practice managed care principles;

- willingness to follow the group's utilization review and quality assurance policies; and
- participation in managed care contracts:
- financial performance:
  - evidence of financial stability in past practice management; and
  - demonstration of productivity and efficiency;
- other:
  - excellent communication skills (e.g., oral and written);
  - good references;
  - appropriate experience level (years in community and practice);
  - sufficient group practice commitment; and
  - acceptability to the founding group members:
    - respect for/by colleagues;
    - team players willing to participate in the group governance process;
    - professional knowledge and expertise;
    - positive employee relations/morale;
    - flexibility and adaptability to change; and
    - ability to work in a capitated reimbursement environment.

Another important requirement for successful medical groups is the proper mix (number and specialties) of physicians to be responsive to the local market, especially in managed care markets. Groups with a large percentage of managed or capitated care are asking for trouble if they have too few primary care physicians or too many specialists. Having the right mix of physicians at the right time with the right quality at the right price is required for medical group competitiveness.

A different physician mix under capitation

National average [2]
(34% primary care)

Capitated system [3]
(65% primary care)

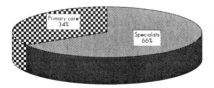
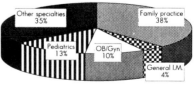

Successful medical groups extensively screen new recruits, using multiple interviews, reference checks as well as in-depth interview checklists. It is impossible for a medical group to spend too much time selecting the right physicians.

Practice profiling

Before completing financial proformas on what it will cost to form a group, it is necessary to profile the practices of individual physicians that will be joining the new group practice. The data developed in this profile process will be very valuable later in the group formation process. It helps design initial group physician compensation formulas and determine whether individual physicians will meet group expectations for productivity, clinical quality, financial stability or other performance standards.

Sources of physician practice profile information

- computer-generated production reports;
- appointment books or computer printouts;
- legal documents and agreements;
- financial statements, records, payroll tax reports and tax returns;
- payer contracts, billing and insurance documentation; and
- leases (office and equipment).

Personnel collecting physician practice profile data should be able to deal effectively with physicians and on-site physician interviews should be conducted or the data collection effort will probably be delayed. The methods for collecting and analyzing data should be disclosed to the physicians under review, and safeguards against unauthorized use or disclosure of the profiles should be developed.

Sample physician practice profile information

- physician productivity (patient encounters, hospital visits, active files);
- patient mix (capitation, fee-for-service, Medicare, Medicaid);
- net revenue generated (charges, collection percentage);
- assets (tangible assets, accounts receivable);
- liabilities (long-term debt, outstanding litigation);
- cost structure (overhead, full-time-employees per physician);
- employee compensation and benefits;
- physician compensation and benefits;
- billing and computer systems;
- managed care and capitation systems;
- facility locations and ownership; and
- other (practice structure, age, certifications, etc.).

Bob Dickinson, of BDC Advisors in San Francisco, cautions against rushing into practice profiling without proper planning and coordination. He outlines nine steps that should be followed to successfully profile physician practices.

Nine steps to successfully profile physician practices [4]

1. Manage physician expectations;

2. Assign a point person;

3. Only request the data that you will use;

4. Manage nonphysician personnel;

5. Get physician buy-in;

6. Distinguish between unavailable versus undisclosed information;

7. Identify key issues/outliers;

8. Be on-site; and

9. Return all originals.

Practice asset valuations

For physicians who are selling their practices to a hospital, health plan or existing group practice, practice profiling is a required step for physician practice valuation. During practice profiling, potential buyers can do appropriate due diligence of each physician practice to determine whether the practices are desirable purchases. In some markets, only tangible assets of physician practices are being purchased by these practice buyers, while in other markets, both tangible and intangible assets are being purchased. Liabilities of physicians may or may not be assumed by the practice buyer, and accounts receivable may or may not be purchased. Nonprofit hospitals and groups have special Internal Revenue Service guidelines and other regulatory requirements as to acceptable methodologies of valuation. For groups being formed solely by physicians, normally a portion of tangible assets and/or cash is contributed to capitalize the group practice in exchange for group stock or partnership interests which may also necessitate valuation of contributed assets.

Practice asset valuation approaches

- income approaches;
  - excess earnings method; and
  - discounted cash flow method;
- market approaches;
  - market comparison method; and
  - comparative transaction method;
- cost approaches;
  - book value; and
  - replacement cost.

Market assessment

The next step in determining the feasibility of forming a group practice is to complete an assessment of the market the group practice serves. This step evaluates possible group competitors as well as develops data for financial proformas on group formation.

Market assessment steps

- definition of the medical group service area;
- projections of potential payer contracts and payer mix;
- interviews of employers and payers;
- analysis of competitive groups and other provider networks; and
- development of target markets.

Initial financial assessment

Before going any further in the group formation process, the financial feasibility of forming a group practice should be determined as well as potential funding sources. Initial financial proformas of the projected capital and operational costs should be developed based on the expected numbers of physicians joining the group. If physician practices are going to be acquired, purchase prices per physician practice should be estimated. For groups formed solely by physicians, physicians interested in joining the group should have clear expectations of their own financial risks and potential capital contributions. Conservative estimates of formation costs should be developed, as inevitably actual costs will exceed projected costs.

PHASE II: BUSINESS PLANNING

Legal structure

The next step in forming a group practice is to determine the legal structure of the group.

Some legal structure alternatives for medical groups

For-profit alternatives	Nonprofit alternatives
• partnership; • professional corporation; • professional corporation aligned with a management services organization; and • limited liability company (in some states).	• "freestanding" medical foundation; • medical foundation aligned with a professional corporation; • medical foundation integrated with a hospital or health system; and • non-equity corporation or limited liability company/nonprofit partners.

Those involved in forming a medical group should *first* decide on their mutual objectives and goals and *then* tailor a structural model to support those objectives and goals.

Considerations for selection of legal structure

- analysis of needs of likely physician participants;
- valuation/compensation/funding sources issues;
- physician considerations/sensitivity in selling/merging practices;
- comparative advantages/disadvantages of available structures; and
- legal and regulatory issues:
    - corporate practice of medicine;
    - fraud and abuse regulations;
    - Stark I and II;
    - private inurement; and
    - federal and state licensing regulations and taxation.

The willingness of physicians to accept a legal structure is a key consideration in its selection. Several questions should be asked before agreeing on a structure: Would physicians mind if another entity holds their managed care contracts? Are physicians unwilling to become employees of a capital partner (hospital, health plan or others)? What role in governance do group physicians want? Are physicians willing to sell all their assets to a capital partner (hospital, health plan or others)? How important to potential group physicians is physician equity in the medical group?

Ownership

Directly related to selecting a legal structure is the determination of ownership of group assets. There is great debate on whether medical group legal structures which include physician equity are ultimately more successful than those that do not. Frequently, physician ownership is a misnomer when group physicians have little or no personal equity invested and others (hospitals, banks, health plans, etc.) have invested or lent the majority of group capital (with appropriate security for their investments or loans). In 1993, the Advisory Board Company, a national research organization, stirred up controversy among its health system membership (which includes many nonprofit, community hospitals) by grading equity models as the most sustainable models for physician-hospital integration.[5] In response, some hospitals have created equity models by forming aligned medical groups with two classes of equity: nominal equity held by physicians, and real equity held by the major capital investor which is usually the hospital.

One of the disadvantages of physician equity in medical groups is the need to require new physicians to buy into the group. This may make it difficult to recruit new group physicians. In addition, medical groups need liquid funds to buy out physicians who leave or pass away. Significant group cash flow problems may occur if a large number of group physicians leave at one time. In addition, conflicts arise if some group physicians have equity and others don't

Governance

Albert Barnett, M.D., chief executive officer of the Friendly Hills Health Care Network in La Habra, Calif., describes the process of selecting a medical group governance body:

> Careful consideration should be given to the size of the executive committee [or board] ... the smaller, the better; the ideal size is perhaps five voting members, with a maximum of seven. Since most physicians feel they have the necessary qualifications

to be effective ... members ... it is often difficult to restrict membership to a small number ...

The committee [or board] generally becomes a microcosm of the entire group ... Once elected, however ... members should act for the benefit of the whole organization and not as representatives of factions within the organization ... members should remember that their duty is to support the mission statement and ensure the continuity of the organization, not to curry favors for their individual coteries. [6]

A group without good governance is a group that will fail. Strong governance requires medical group boards to take an oversight and policy role with appropriate delegation to management, excellent communication among all parties, and collaborative decision making between both physician and administrative leaders.

When medical groups are small, decisions may be made by the entire physician membership. It is imperative for these groups to evolve into using an executive committee or a board of directors to avoid being bogged down in micro-management. In most medical groups, boards are exclusively composed of physicians; however, this is changing as medical groups are affiliating with other capital partners.

The process of selecting a board as well as the board's responsibilities should be clearly articulated. Terms of board members should be structured to allow continuity yet eventual board turnover (staggered three to six year terms). Board candidates should meet standards for qualification based on leadership competencies.

Physician compensation

Probably the most controversial and difficult part of forming a medical group is getting a consensus on the physician compensation plan to be used. Medical groups have the same issues in determining how the pie is to be split as other organizations of professionals (accountants, attorneys, architects, etc.) and there are as many ways of determining compensation as there are medical groups.

Before setting out to develop a group compensation plan, it is important to survey the historical compensation methodologies of the founding physicians of the medical group. If the initial medical group compensation plan will result in drastic changes in how these physicians are compensated (especially if their compensation or benefits will go down), then these physicians will probably not support it. One alternative is to use historical compensation methodologies for these founding physicians in the first year of the new group practice.

Survey of historical compensation of founding physicians

- Determine historical compensation methods;
- Examine five-year earnings and benefits history;
- Review unusual historical arrangements (unpaid working spouses, no employee benefits, outside income, administrative compensation);
- List historical payers, payer mix; and
- Review of historical individual physician performance:
  - collections (volume, collection ratio, accounts receivable aging);
  - encounter complexity (Medicare, hospital);
  - productivity (patient visits, number of patients, enrollees, hours, billings);
  - efficiency (utilization, risk-pool sharing, overhead, etc.); and
  - discretionary performance (quality, patient satisfaction, etc.).

Susan Cejka, president of Cejka & Company in St. Louis, Mo., recommends establishing two primary objectives of a group compensation plan: (1) to enhance the ability of the organization to achieve its long-term goals, and (2) to distribute available group cash fairly and appropriately.

Primary objectives of a medical group compensation plan [7]

Achieve long-term group goals	Distribute cash fairly and appropriately
• Ensure financial viability of the group; • Promote harmony within the group; • Account for competitive environment; • Enhance organizational environment; • Support M.D. recruitment and retention; and • Encourage the efficient and effective practice of medicine.	• Distribute income in accordance with effort and contribution; • Distribute cash in accordance with sources of revenue; and • Account for built-in biases.

Compensation plans should be simple to understand and include incentives to foster the success of the medical group. In order for compensation formulas to be fair, different levels of service by medical group physicians need to be accounted for (such as the differences between service for young capitated patients vs. elderly Medicare patients).

Compensation plan alternatives [8]

- production formulas:
- Individual production formulas reward physicians in direct relationship to the revenue they produce; and
- Equal share formulas split the excess of revenue over expenses among group members evenly. These plans are designed to build group culture, values and teamwork;
- salary formulas:
- Indexed salary plans rely on comparisons to standard benchmarks for a prescribed scope of work, with annual increases linked to merit or time of service; and
- Market-based salary and bonus plans seek to balance the stability of a salary with incentive payments to stimulate desired behaviors. The plans often include some elements of a production formula;
- capitation formulas:
- Capitation formulas assign the responsibilities associated with meeting the goals of managed care contracts to the physicians directly;
- Gatekeeper formulas assign the main task of managing care to the primary care providers; and
- Department or individual capitation formulas assign a specific scope of risk to each physician involved in the delivery of care.

Capitation or salary compensation formulas should be developed as the percentage of a medical group's capitation business expands. Using traditional production compensation formulas in a capitated medical group usually results in poor medical group financial performance. Medical groups should customize their capitation compensation plans based on the physician behaviors they want to reward. That includes patient satisfaction, high quality and efficient medicine.

Medical group capitation formulas

- physician capitation options;
  - primary care capitation, specialists fee-for-service;
  - primary care fee-for-service, specialists capitation;
  - capitation of primary care and specialists; and
  - capitation by specialty or individual physician;
- physician salary options;
  - salary from all revenue sources — fee-for-service and capitation;
  - salary from only capitation revenue sources; and
  - salary plus bonus;
- physician discretionary income or bonuses; and
- any combination of the above.

As medical group compensation plans evolve, they should reduce individual physician risk and include incentives to meet group performance objectives (e.g., quality, patient satisfaction, efficiency, productivity, etc.), rather than individual performance objectives.

Evolution of physician compensation plans [9]

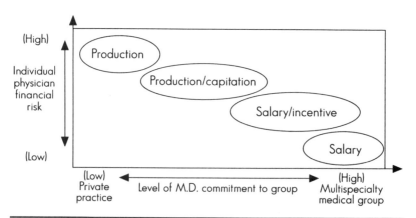

Physician work effort standards

In their formation, many groups overlook the establishment of standards for physician work effort in order to maintain an efficient and viable medical group operation. This is a very sensitive subject with physicians, because many consider it demeaning to their profession to have someone tracking their productivity. However, not all physicians give equal effort, and it is critical that medical groups have realistic tracking mechanisms to reward those physicians who are productive. This is important even in a capitated medical group in which the productive physician can manage more enrollees while maintaining quality, service and efficiency.

Measurement of physician work effort	
Components measured	**Measurement approaches**
• allocations of physician time (call, administrators, hospital, other); • patient visits by physician (adjusted for patient mix); • collections, billings by physician (adjusted for source of payment); • number of patients, enrollees by physician (adjusted for patient/ enrollee mix); and • hours worked by physician.	• tracking of patient appointments kept; • tracking of managed care enrollees and/or medical charts by physician (adjusted for patient/ enrollee mix); • accounting of collections, billings by physician (adjusted for source of payment); and • physician time sheets or other tracking mechanisms of physician time (adjusted for patient mix).

Business plan and budgets

A five-year business plan should be prepared for a new medical group with related annual operating and capital budgets. The business plan should incorporate the results of the market assessment completed above as well as several other considerations:

Business plan inclusions

- expected levels of patient care and managed care services by the medical group;
- number of anticipated practice sites and their capital and operating requirements;
- projected physician and other professional staffing requirements;
- the type and scope of ancillary services, if any, to be operated by the medical group;
- the anticipated costs of recruitment and other practice development expenses;
- specific marketing, managed care and other strategies to maintain and enhance marketshare;
- sources and uses of cash; and
- priorities of the medical group as to equipment and other capital requirements.

**Examples of business plan
and budget principles**

- Meet business plan and budget targets for the medical group;
  - financial profit by year four;
  - accumulation of reserves at agreed upon rate by year four;
  - no addition of debt beyond amounts specified in the business plan;
- Generate sufficient revenues to pay a reasonable return to capital investors and return the initial capital investment over an agreed upon time frame; and
- Generate sufficient margins to provide market competitive compensation for the medical group physicians.

Legal documents

Before a medical group can become official, several legal documents should be prepared and executed. The types of documents depend on the legal structure selected for the medical group.

Examples of medical group formation legal documents

Partnership	Professional corporation	Medical foundation	Limited liability company
• partnership agreement; • buy-sell agreement; and • employment agreements.	• articles of incorporation; • bylaws; • employment agreements; and • stock purchase and redemption agreement.	• articles of incorporation; • bylaws; • professional services agreement; and • employment agreements.	• articles of incorporation; • operating agreement; and • employment agreement.

Legal documents should reflect the principles and values of the parties forming the medical group, not determine them. Competent, experienced legal advice should be sought in developing group formation legal documents.

PHASE III: PRE-IMPLEMENTATION

Management

Determining the management team for a new medical group is an important step in the formation process. Depending on the size of the medical group, there may be one or several managers, an administrator and a medical director, and there may also be a physician president/CEO.

Key areas of medical group management [10]	
• top-level management;	• medical records;
• patient care management;	• legal matters and contracting;
• operations;	• management information systems;
• finance;	• marketing;
• quality assurance;	• recruitment and retention of staff;
• risk management;	• human resources;
• medical and surgical utilization review;	• managed care management; and
• peer review;	• education and training.

Robert Nelson, former executive director of the Harriman Jones Medical Group in Long Beach, Calif., describes the role of the medical group administrator:

> There are few administrative jobs more complex than managing a medical group ... At the same time, a medical group uses highly trained professionals as production workers, professionals who have never been educated in fundamental business practices.
>
> The need for strong management is evident. But strong management does not consist of independent actions ... The management of a medical group in the 1990s must be a team effort, and the role of the medical group administrator is to be a part of the management team.
>
> In the sophisticated and complex medical marketplace of the 1990s, there is probably no medical group that should not have at least one full-time administrator. Each administrator should be skilled in business and finance. Medicine is no longer simply a profession of service to patients in which only simple supervision is required. [11]

Robert Nelson describes a recommended list of responsibilities defining the administrator's role (see Appendix A). Medical groups must be careful in designing the interface between group medical directors and administrators, and should also define the group medical director's role (see Appendix A).

> To avoid two management systems, one for physicians and one for nonphysician staff, the medical directorship is treated as a staff rather than a line position. It is essentially a facilitating and advisory position, and no staff members directly report to the medical director . . . The medical director has jurisdiction over the medical staff . . . quality assurance and peer review . . . there must be an advisory link. [12]

Allocation of decision making and responsibilities

If the new medical group is aligned with a medical foundation or a management services organization, decision making and re-sponsibilities must be allocated to each entity (the medical group and the lay entity). The California Medical Association commissioned a study group to provide recommendations on allocations of deci-sion making and responsibilities. The results of this study follow:

Allocation of decision making authority [13]

	Medical group makes ultimate decision
Exclusive (medical group)	• setting purely medical practice policies; • deciding what conditions can be referred to another physician specialist; • deciding what diagnostic tests are appropriate for a particular condition; • deciding what gets included in a particular patient's medical record; • deciding whether a particular patient visit requires a particular billing code; • communicating with patients; and • determining whether an emergency exists.
Consultative (w/lay partner)	• determining practice parameters; • making treatment decisions that involve bioethical issues; • credentialing for specific procedures and setting general standards as applied to individuals; • scheduling on-call coverage; • handling impaired physicians; and • deciding which CME courses should be taken.

	Medical group makes ultimate decision
Shared (w/lay partner)	• allocating resources; • establishing bioethics policies; • deciding the types of technologies that should be employed; • deciding to whom a physician can refer a patient; • establishing standards for admission to the medical group; • deciding on individual applicants for admission to the group; • developing, implementing and enforcing UR and QA plans; • determining whether to consider an application for admission; • selecting independent "limited license practitioners" and "physician extenders," and deciding whether and when to use extenders; • developing drug formularies; • selecting key medical officers; controlling medical data; and • deciding how many patients a physician should see.
	Medical group and lay partner make shared decision
Joint decisions (both medical group and lay partner)	• deciding how many hours a physician should work; • making non-clinical decisions concerning medical records; • entering contractual relationships with third-party payers; • deciding level and scope of malpractice coverage; • deciding physician compensation policies and parameters; • settling cases for all parties named in an action; • marketing; • setting the global budget for all physician and limited license practitioner compensation; • establishing grievance policies; • making a decision to transfer a patient; • dealing with mergers, acquisitions, conversions and affiliations; • deciding ownership and scope of ancillary services; • deciding level of indigent care provided; and • deciding employment matters.
	Lay partner makes ultimate decision
Exclusive (lay partner)	• determining compensation for allied health and lay staff; and • selecting purely administrative staff that do not hold key positions.
Consultative (w/med grp)	• coding and billing procedures; and • controlling administrative data.
Shared (w/med grp)	• selecting nonphysician dependent practitioners only; • selecting key administrators; • purchasing, replacing and repairing equipment; and • deciding how much patients should pay.

Even though different entities are responsible for different decisions, it is important that all decisions be made based on the consensus of all parties.

Building consensus [14]

- broadening the base of organizational ownership;
- sharing and communicating company goals to all members;
- expanding leadership responsibilities and empowerment;
- maintaining a policy of fairness and honesty with all group members; and
- facilitating free and open communication among the leadership and all group members.

Roles and responsibilities of each entity must also be defined: [15]

Role of lay partner	Role of medical groups
• clinic premises; • utilities, building services, supplies; • equipment, furniture; • repairs and maintenance; • new equipment; • administrative and nonphysician staff; • accounting, billing, collections; • managed care contracts; • financial management and reports; • marketing and public relations; • management information systems; and • corporate support services.	• employment; • professional supervision and training; • physician compensation; • criteria and selection of physicians; • quality and utilization management; • professional evaluation of clinic; • capital budget initiation; • all patient care decisions; and • all decisions on physician staffing, scheduling.

Practice merger proposals

When physician practices are acquired or merged as part of the medical group formation process, asset merger proposals should be developed. Physicians should clearly understand the assets and liabilities they will retain and transfer to the new group. Legal documents may reflect provisions for repurchase or return of assets should an individual physician terminate employment.

Sample physician practice merger proposal [16]

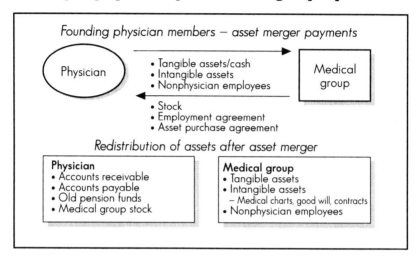

Founding physician members – asset merger payments

Physician

- Tangible assets/cash
- Intangible assets
- Nonphysician employees

- Stock
- Employment agreement
- Asset purchase agreement

Medical group

Redistribution of assets after asset merger

Physician
- Accounts receivable
- Accounts payable
- Old pension funds
- Medical group stock

Medical group
- Tangible assets
- Intangible assets
  – Medical charts, good will, contracts
- Nonphysician employees

Site planning

To improve economies of scale and generate ancillary revenues, medical groups should consolidate office sites while maintaining patient convenience and access. A site plan should be prepared as part of the business planning process based on analysis of the medical group's service area (patient demographics, physician supply and demand, payers and payer mix, etc.).

Existing physician sites should be evaluated for possible use. The cost of assuming current leases and potential capital outlays for new land and facilities should be estimated. Some physicians may have to dispose of facilities or sublet them. A dynamic work plan anticipating the timing of moves should be outlined, with plenty of room for error. Physicians involved should clearly understand that they may be expected to move, and that office consolidations are not an option (group practices without walls are unable to achieve economies of scale).

Genesis Healthcare International, Inc. has outlined a series of preferred characteristics associated with a model primary care physician practice site. These guidelines, listed below, should be adapted for local market conditions:

Model primary care physician practice site [17]

- Hours of operation: 8 a.m. to 8 p.m.

- Physician mix: The ideal mix is to have four to six primary care physicians (family practitioner, general internist and pediatrician) in each center. Additional physicians should be added to a given center in multiples of this mix (e.g., a larger center would have eight to 12 physicians with the same specialty [mix]).

- Physician assistants/nurse practitioners: The use of these professionals will increase. Current discussions with physicians suggest that an appropriate ratio of physicians to physician extenders will be one to one by 1998. Each center should be developed to accommodate the increased use of these professionals in the future.

- Geographic distribution: Primary care centers should be located within 5 miles or a 15-minute drive from the customer. The point of reference for the customer could be either the worksite or the home.

Implementation plan

The final step in forming a medical group is to develop an implementation plan. At this point, the group vision and guiding principles should be articulated; the initial physicians who will be joining the group identified; the physician compensation plan agreed to; governance, ownership and management identified; legal documents completed and executed; a market assessment and business plan prepared and approved; asset merger proposals and valuations finalized; and a preliminary site plan completed. The implementation plan builds on all these steps, and establishes time lines and responsible parties to start medical group operations. Each medical group will have a unique implementation plan depending on local market conditions and group composition (see Appendix B for an example of a medical group implementation plan).

PHASE IV: IMPLEMENTATION

Successful implementation of a new medical group requires appropriate education, communication and planning. Physicians joining a new group must clearly understand the process involved and the timing of each step. Neither Rome nor medical groups can be built in a day. All parties must work together as a team to properly execute the implementation plan.

Office consolidation

For medical groups that are being formed with a collection of existing solo practices, there will normally be a time lag until practices can be consolidated. Existing physician office leases must occasionally be honored, new facilities constructed (six months to 18 months), and existing systems and personnel transitioned. It is critical that physicians joining a new group understand the expectations of the group concerning the need for and timing of office consolidation. Sometimes the group may want a physician to move to an underserved or high-demand location. Another factor to be aware of is potential staff attrition due to the uncertainty of personnel changes. To have a smooth office consolidation, communication with all affected parties is key. Also, the medical group should be sensitive to the compensation impact of required relocations, and take appropriate steps to assure fair treatment of all group members during this transition period.

Operations

An administrator should be hired quickly after the group is formed to implement operational systems and procedures. The already-developed medical group implementation plan should be used as a basis for establishing operations with the administrator, understanding the need to be flexible in following the plan. The new group administrator should draw on the experiences of others. Excellent resources are available from Medical Group Management Association (MGMA) for every area of medical group operations.

Management information systems (MIS)

A big mistake frequently made in forming new medical groups is to rush the decision for a new, expensive computer system. If solo practices are going to be combined to form a new group, invariably the best way to start the group is to use one or more of the existing systems available rather than start from scratch with a completely new system. Professional advice should be sought from MIS consultants. A careful review of medical group needs and MIS vendors and products should be done. Many problems will be avoided later on if the management information system is allowed to evolve over time. Sometimes manual systems are very effective in the early stages of a new medical group and can serve to develop confidence of medical group personnel as the medical group transitions to more comprehensive, computerized solutions.

Percentage of medical groups that have or plan to have management information systems, 1995 [18]

Size (# of full-time physicians)	Have computer-ized medical records	Plan to computer-ize medical records	Have automated appoint-ment scheduling	Plan to automate appoint-ment scheduling
10 or Fewer	15.6%	74.7%	41.8%	58.4%
11-25	21.7%	82.6%	52.6%	80.0%
26-50	6.7%	73.3%	76.9%	100.0%
51-100	7.1%	100.0%	45.5%	100.0%
101 or more	7.1%	100.0%	61.5%	100.0%
Specialty compostion:				
Single specialty	16.4%	75.5%	42.5%	57.6%
Multispecialty	10.1%	79.9%	47.2%	76.7%
All groups	15.4%	75.1%	43.4%	60.3%

Managed care systems

For those groups that have a large percentage of capitated or managed care patients, it is critical that effective systems be developed to track and control managed care costs. In addition, payers are increasingly expecting providers to demonstrate not only lower prices, but documented quality service and care as well as good outcomes. Medical groups should have at least one physician assigned to work with the medical group administrator in developing and implementing utilization review and quality assurance programs.

Contracting and marketing

Effective contracting and marketing systems and procedures are essential for medical groups to enhance their patient base and marketshare. A managed care contracting strategy should be developed and implemented for the medical group. Marketing programs should be developed that build on the medical group's identity and each physician's reputation. Relationships with payers should be developed and market opportunities identified. The best marketing is, of course, providing high quality service at a low cost.

A new marketing approach

'New' medical group marketing:	'Old' medical group marketing:
• community- and patient-focused; • appropriate geographic coverage, size; • adequate and proper mix of physicians; • high quality, cost-effective services; • accessible, convenient locations; • demonstrated added value in the market.	• internal- and physician-focused; • limited geographic coverage, size; • inappropriate mix of physicians; • expensive, low quality services; • inaccessible, inconvenient locations; and • no differentiated value in the market.

Notes

[1] "Integrated Health Care: Reorganizing the Physician, Hospital and Health Plan Relationship," Coddington, Moore and Fischer, 1994, p. 113.

[2] "Physician Characteristics and Distribution in the U.S.," American Medical Association, 1993.

[3] "Organizing to Manage Risk," *Integrated Healthcare Report*, May 1993.

[4] "Developing A Primary Care Group Practice: Getting Started," *Medical Staff Strategy Report*, 1993.

[5] "The Grand Alliance — Vertical Strategies for Physicians and Health Systems," The Advisory Board Company, 1993.

[6] "Ambulatory Care Management and Practice, Edited by A. Barnett, M.D. and G. Mayer, RN, EdD, FAAN, p. 17.

[7] Ibid., p. 77,

[8] Ibid.

[9] A presentation to Gould Medical Group, Modesto, Calif., by Ed Baloun, Executive Consulting Group, Inc., Seattle, Wash., 1992.

[10] "Ambulatory Care Management and Practice, Edited by A. Barnett, M.D. and G. Mayer, RN, EdD, FAAN, p. 20.

[11] Ibid., pp. 53-55.

[12] Ibid., p. 27.

[13] "Dimensions of Control," *Integrated Healthcare Report*, September 1992.

[14] *Ambulatory Care Management and Practice*, Edited by A. Barnett, M.D. and G. Mayer, RN, EdD, FAAN, p. 12.

[15] "Dimensions of Control," *Integrated Healthcare Report*, September, 1992.

[16] A presentation by Richard Wessland, BDC Advisors Healthcare Consulting Firm, San Francisco, Calif., at a national conference on forming medical groups, 1993.

[17] LMC Ambulatory Services Strategic Plan, Genesis Healthcare International, Inc., 1994, p. 40.

[18] Holchst Marion Roussel, Inc., *Medical Group Practice Digest*, 1995, p. 26.

PART TWO

The Management of Medical Groups

Several medical groups in this country are well run, efficient, growing, profitable and successful. Unfortunately, these groups sometimes appear to be in the minority. Far too many groups struggle to manage effectively, especially as they grow. As medicine goes through the shake-out that several other U.S. businesses have already experienced, medical groups are prime candidates for restructuring.

Various organizations are springing up around the country to attempt to seize the profit opportunities created by ineffective management of medical groups. Some of these organizations affiliate with physicians and medical groups primarily to generate anticipated profits available from such affiliations (physician management companies, health systems, health plans, etc.). Other organizations affiliate with physicians for different motives, such as creating true integrated delivery systems to serve their communities. If physicians in medical groups do not choose their partners wisely, they and their profits will be "owned" and "controlled" by others.

Management of medical groups is an art not a science. Concepts of how to manage medical groups are constantly evolving, and need to adapt to the changing health care environment. The following ideas on ways to better manage medical groups are humbly presented with the knowledge that they could become obsolete rather quickly.

Medical group administrators and managers have challenging and exciting jobs. As health care transitions from a hospital focus to an ambulatory care and physician focus, opportunities abound for effective medical group managers. In their roles they must wear several hats: psychologists, accountants, negotiators, salespeople, etc. They need to be versatile in their approaches to problem solving and tough under fire. Their jobs are more difficult when they have to both manage physicians as medical group employees and report to the same physicians in their roles as medical group board members and owners. Managing independently minded physicians has been described as being as difficult as "herding cats."

A few years ago, few physicians were in medical group management positions. More and more physicians are obtaining training and experience to become medical group managers. They are leading the way in providing innovative ideas for managing medical groups.

The following discussion critically examines some management problems medical groups are experiencing and offers suggestions on simple improvements that most medical groups can make. These problems are broken down into four general areas: organization and governance; medical group economics; physician compensation and benefits; and medical group operations.

Those medical groups that have avoided the majority of these problems are the strongest groups. Those that have a predominance of these problems (as well as other problems) may be in jeopardy of collapsing. As physician and administrative leaders accept responsibility for managing medical groups, it is important for them to have a clear vision of the challenges ahead.

CHAPTER FIVE

Organization and Governance

Medical group culture

An important ingredient in successful medical groups is development of a group culture. Frederick Wenzel, executive director and CEO of Medical Group Management Association, describes what group culture is:

> [Group] culture has been defined in a variety of ways, but its most useful definition comes down to the "way we do things." It has also been described as a system of shared beliefs, values and behaviors within an organization. Like mercury, it is elusive. [Group] culture exists implicitly. It is both ubiquitous and unnoticed. Authors ... suggest that [group] culture consists of the norms, values and unwritten rules of conduct within an organization together with its management style, priorities, beliefs and interpersonal behaviors. [1]

Many medical groups are really just collections of independent, solo practices agreeing to share expenses. They do not have the cohesiveness to hold together if times get tough. Indicators that a group culture does not exist are obvious in many medical groups.

Evidence that a medical group lacks culture

Physicians are:
- unwilling to delegate authority or give up individual autonomy;
- unable to work collaboratively to solve problems;
- not committed to or willing to follow group goals and directives;
- refusing to move towards consolidation of practices and true economies of scale;
- unwilling to share income, expense or governance;
- focused on the short-term, not the long-term; and
- unwilling to deal with problems with other group physicians.

Medical group cultures are not built overnight. They are very dependent on the makeup of the physician members of the medical group. As described in *The Physician Group Practice*:

> For successful participation in group practice requires, in addition to specialized competence in some field of medicine, certain very special traits of character without which a man [woman] is likely to be unhappy in this type of practice. The most essential characteristic is dedication — unselfish dedication to the ideal of providing the best medical care — and when a man [woman] has this trait, such undesirable qualities as avarice and envy do not exist. The next most important characteristic for a group member is professional competence. This is important of course in every physician, but it is essential in a group member because the acts of one member reflect so acutely on the status of the whole group... A group member must be capable of teamwork; he [she] must be able to adjust with flexibility and amiability to the personalities of his [her] associates, diverse though they may be. It is lack of this ability, rigid individualism so to speak, which is the most common failure of a man [woman] to make a success of group practice ... And finally, the physician going into group practice must have a deep sense of loyalty to his [her] fellows in the group and to the group as an institution. [2]

Medical groups should follow certain steps to ensure they develop an appropriate group culture.

Steps to develop a medical group culture

- The first step in establishing a group culture is to have the "right" physicians with the "right" shared vision. Without physicians who support a shared vision, no matter what other steps a medical group takes, "group-think" will never happen. The shared vision should be group-oriented, not individual-oriented, and understood and embraced by all group physicians. Group goals and objectives should be developed based of this vision, and tracking mechanisms should ensure that the group meets these goals and objectives.
- Development of an effective governance structure is the next priority. A small-sized board or executive committee should be formally nominated and elected with clear differentiation between the roles of the board (policy-making) and management (policy-implementation).
- Finally, strong leadership (both physician and administrative) must be in place for success. This leadership must be given appropriate accountabilities and group delegation of authority. Roles and responsibilities should be well understood and leaders should be selected based on competence.

Combining the "right physicians" with the "right vision," the "right governance" and the "right leadership" is the key to developing a successful group culture.

The importance of governance

Most medical group problems stem from inadequate group governance.

> Group practices in particular are remarkably similar to college fraternities. Individual freedom of expression is the central driving force. Each person is highly committed to selfish special interests. The primary reason for being together is not task interdependence.
>
> Individual member commitment is time-bounded (e.g., four years at college). Dues will be paid as long "as I get what I want." This fraternity orientation feeds, and is consistent with, a mind set of low tolerance for delayed gratification ... Goodies — such as money, time off and trips to professional development meetings in Hawaii and Bermuda — like food on the frat dinner table, are grabbed by those with the longest reach and quickest hands. [3]

Without effective governance, medical groups are candidates for significant performance problems and potential eventual breakup. Poorly governed medical groups usually have the following characteristics in common:

Evidence of poor medical group governance

- physicians are part-time, untrained micro-managers;
- individual physicians are valued more than the group;
- deviant individual physician behavior is tolerated for some time;
- decision making is consensual and delayed;
- the most popular, not the most competent, leaders are selected;
- physician leader self-interest (not group-interest) dictates decisions; and
- management delegation is difficult or nonexistent.

The medical groups around the United States that are the most successful usually have strong governance. Long-established medical groups may fall into decay when strong, founding physician leaders retire or pass away.

Evidence of strong medical group governance

- shared vision of group goals and objectives;
- established and followed group principles;
- effective and competent physician and administrative leadership;
- appropriate delegation of authority to management;
- group orientation, not individual orientation;
- business and strategic plans with follow up; and
- policy-making medical group board.

Physician leadership

Related to inadequate group governance is the lack of enough "trained physician leaders." The most successful medical groups have developed "key physician leaders" in their governance structures since nonphysician administrators or managers, at least in the current environment, are not considered "equal" to physicians by group physicians. "As one physician-administrator at the Carle Clinic said, 'I am not in this job because of my administrative skills.' Although he has an M.B.A. degree, he said, 'I am effective because I am a physician and have the respect of my fellow doctors.'" [4] James Farrell and Morley Robbins, of the Hay Group, describe the need for physician leadership in the 1990s:

> At no point in the history of organized medicine has there been a greater need for physician leadership ... the role of the physician, as core provider, is undergoing significant re-evaluation and adjustment. Trained to be individual experts and independent decision makers, physicians now find themselves thrust into group problem solving and collaborative decision making. [5]

As more and more physicians accept management roles in medical groups, they need to learn new skills and competencies. M. McCall and J. Clair, of the University of Southern California Graduate School of Business Administration, state that "the doctor manager is the epitome of the oxymoron, for never in the history of language have two terms been so utterly opposed." [6] McCall and Clair go on to list 10 deadly flaws that cause physician managers to fail:

10 reasons why physician managers fail [7]

1. Insensitivity and arrogance;
2. Inability to choose staff;
3. Over managing (inability to delegate);
4. Inability to adapt to a superior;
5. Fighting the wrong battles;
6. Being seen as untrustworthy (having questionable motives);
7. Failing to develop a strategic vision;
8. Being overwhelmed by the job;
9. Lacking specific management skills or knowledge; and
10. Lacking commitment to the job.

Many physician leaders are very competent and do outstanding jobs for their medical groups. The most prestigious medical groups in this country are generally headed by well qualified and respected physician leaders. Several physicians are obtaining advanced degrees in management and valuable on-the-job leadership experience. Albert Barnett, M.D., describes the transition group medical directors have had to make:

> In the past, physicians elected or appointed to the role of medical director had virtually no background in management or administration. In small or emerging group practices, such individuals might have been group founders who desired to cut back on their clinical duties ... Often they were older physicians who had benign personalities and were unlikely to interfere ... Today, the role of medical director is dramatically different, especially in large group practices and in groups with a large stake in prepaid managed care ... This shift to managerial and administrative functions for the medical director has caught many groups off guard, leaving them forced to contend with physician managers who possess the wrong or inadequate skills in an increasingly competitive arena. [8]

Farrell and Robbins describe several important leadership competencies that medical group physician leaders should possess. Leadership competencies for a medical group physician president/CEO are listed on the next page.

Physician leadership competencies [9]

Leadership competencies	Example: Medical group president
• Strategic business orientation	• Effectively positions the group within the delivery system and the market
• Empowering/developing others	• Empowers others to accomplish strategic goals
• Mission articulation	• Acts as a champion to define and promote organizations mission
• Group leadership	• Develops cooperative and collaborative working relationships
• Negotiation skills	• Demonstrates ability to forge strategic relationships and agreements to further the organization's mission
• Stakeholder relationship building	• Develops close relationships and strategic linkages
• Organizational awareness	• Maintains intuitive understanding of system dynamics

Problems with medical groups developing physician leaders

- Medical group reluctance to allocate a portion of physician distributable income for compensation of physician and administrative leadership;
- Individual physician concerns about transitioning to leadership roles and potentially losing patients, compensation and practices;
- The gap between administrative salaries and physician salaries;
- The typical medical group orientation towards reduction in current group overhead, rather than investment for long-term group success;
- Inadequate physician educational preparation for leadership roles;
- The expense of appropriate physician leadership development programs;
- The insecurity of any physician leadership position in a medical group;
- The best physician does not necessarily make the best leader; and
- The "I'm a physician, why do I need training?" phenomenon

Medical groups should commit resources to develop physician leaders or "others" will eventually govern them — not necessarily all that bad, just difficult for physicians in most medical groups to swallow.

As stated by Albert Barnett, M.D., "Leadership in a medical group must be based on credibility, fairness and a strong consensus of support. Upon these building blocks are added all the desirable characteristics of leadership."

Physician organizational experience

According to Group Practice Management, Incorporated, Columbia, Mo.,one of the reasons physicians have difficulty governing medical groups is their organizational experience:

> In private ... group medical practice, the physicians themselves are owners of what frequently amounts to a good-sized business organization. The inside exposure of most physicians to good-sized business organizations is limited to universities and hospitals — both of which are customarily large, not-for-profit organizations. It really shows! Perhaps non-profit organizations can afford the luxuries of wheel-spinning committees, indecision, procrastination, petty jealously and gossip. For-profit, private medical groups cannot afford these luxuries, nor can they be organized in a like manner.
>
> Our experiences with groups uncovered an inordinate amount of physician time wasted in non-productive committee work and group meetings. We found groups of 12 and 15 physicians where absolutely no responsibility was delegated below the level of the whole group. Twelve or 15 doctors, if you can imagine, sitting around a table for an hour of heated and indecisive debate about the job performance of Gertrude, the insurance clerk. Or picture the expense committee of six skilled surgeons, spending two hours of their valuable operating room time every week pouring over ... the long distance call to Yakima on August 28. The call cost $2.58, but the doctors spent over $200 [each] of lost time discussing it and concluded by instructing the administrator to check it out. [10]

Physician members of medical groups should come to the realization that responsibilities should be delegated to competent administrators, physician leaders and subordinates. It is impossible for every group physician to participate in every group decision.

Ineffective group managers

One of the biggest problems facing medical groups is ineffective managers. Group Practice Management, Incorporated, discusses some experiences:

> Usually, we could trace the ineffectiveness to simple incompetence or to insecurity. Incompetence will be discussed later. Insecurity, when not coincident with self-realized incompetence, was usually a direct result of the realization that "he [she] had to please everybody." There is no way, of course, to please everybody, but the administrator [or manager], who finds himself [herself] in a group where "everybody has a voice in all decisions" has only two alternatives: correct the group's organizational misconceptions (and risk his [or her] job), or stand patiently by as the foot-servant to the mob and do nothing while the debate goes on (resulting usually in a decision to postpone the decision)."

Robert Nelson describes educational opportunities for medical group managers:

> Continuing education and management networking is essential for managers if they are to keep abreast of the business complexities of modern medicine ... Various associations offer a broad spectrum of educational seminars and courses of study ... Medical Group Management Association (MGMA) ... offers between 50 and 75 educational programs each year aimed at almost every level of experience ... For personal development, the American College of Medical Practice Executives (ACMPE) offers uniquely focused and challenging educational opportunities and assessment tools. [12]

Medical groups with significant managed and capitated care have access to educational tools available through Unified Medical Group Association. Physicians in medical group management can also take advantage of excellent educational programs offered by the American College of Physician Executives.

H.R. Heberlein, in *The Physician Group Practice*, describes several qualifications that medical group managers (or administrators) should have to be effective:

> A manager [administrator] should have a good formal education. Probably the most fitting training, by and large, is business administration, including among other subjects, finance, accounting, commercial law, personnel, public relations, selling, office management, money and banking, insurance, statistics, credit,

purchasing, organization, efficiency studies, communication, public speaking, building, real estate and, certainly, the humanities.

A manager [administrator] must be a leader and a diplomat. He [she] must be pleasant and sincere in his [her] personal relations with those with whom he [she] comes in contact. He [she] must be in complete sympathy with the philosophy of group practice of medicine and in tune with, and have a deep regard for, the high ideals of the medical profession. He [she] should have the capacity and the desire for self-improvement ... [13]

There are some excellent medical group managers who contribute far more to their groups than many of their physicians realize. There are not good benchmarks to judge their skills. Sometimes effective medical group managers and administrators do not work out because the medical group physicians are not interested in making the needed changes they are recommending.

Medical groups should take their time in finding a competent administrator (with medical group management experience), and pay competitive market-based administrative compensation. Medical Group Management Association has an administrator placement service as well as an annual survey of administrator compensation based on group size.

Differences between physicians and administrators

Medical group physicians and administrators have very different experience bases, characteristics and views of the world. Some medical groups have difficulty reconciling these differences, which is why some medical groups have a new administrator every year.

[Administrators] relate to other individuals and groups with an understanding of systems and common goals. On the other hand, physicians are usually individualists. The physician's main relationship to other individuals and groups is primarily a herd behavior, grouping with others of the same kind, with the goal of protecting the individuality of each member of the herd ... These conflicting characteristics make it difficult for [administrators] and practicing physicians to appreciate each other's worlds. [14]

Different characteristics — physicians and administrators [15]

Physician characteristics	Administrator characteristics
• Trained in and concerned with anatomy and/or physiology, diagnosis and treatment of illness and injury. • Often appears to believe that there is no higher authority. • Case-oriented. Concerned with what happens to an individual ... impact of decisions and actions on the welfare of patients. • Gloria Patri thinking. "As it was in the beginning, is now and ever shall be." • Little experience with planning and limiting expenditures. • Fears being disenfranchised. "Don't do anything without asking me first." • May view suggestions about how to practice medicine, or other matters, as "interference" with a physician's "prerogative." • Allegiance is primarily to other practitioners.	• Trained in and concerned with financial matters, group process, personnel management, legalities. • Understands that executive privilege is limited by higher authority. • Data-oriented. Concerned with what happens to groups of patients ... impact of decisions and actions on the goals of the organization. • Responsible for implementing change [skilled at planning for the future]. • Must stay within budget, or control costs to maximize profit. • Delegates responsibilities; go do it and report back. • Expects to be evaluated. Welcomes constructive suggestions that result in improved performance and goal accomplishment. • Allegiance is primarily to the organization.

Dr. Raymond Fernandez, medical director of the Nalle Clinic, describes the difficulty he had transitioning to medical group administration:

> In making the transition from physician to medical director and CEO, I crossed the invisible line between being us and being them ... No matter how hard the physicians try to cover up their feelings, to them I am clearly a traitor ... I tried to strike a compromise by keeping one foot in my practice and one in administration. I even tried maintaining the old call schedule for a while. But before long, I realized that this compromise was not workable ...
>
> Realizing that I had no formal training in business, leadership, management or organizational psychology heightened my personal insecurity ... With no guidelines for measuring success

or predicting the long-term consequences my decisions would have on me and on the group, I had a strong sense of failure ...

I also had to learn to deal with isolation. In this organizational culture that had not had someone in a role of power and authority, physicians have trouble communicating with me. Their view of me as a traitor has shut off certain channels. They neither understand nor appreciate my new role, although they apparently sense that it is essential. I have a related problem with some of the administrators because, as CEO, I am now their boss. They, too, think a physician in an administrative role is a waste: administrators should administer, and physicians should treat patients ...

However, the manager's role has significant differences. I don't see the results of a decision until some time after I've made it. Frequently, my colleagues ask me to tell them what they need to do, which sometimes translates into my telling them how to conduct their practice, but which they see as my telling them how to treat patients ...

In the role of physician-executive, we are supposed to have a clear vision of what is best for our organizations and where to lead them. The simple truth is that we don't really know. Yet to keep our positions as effective leaders, we've got to keep telling our troops where we are taking them. [16]

The different characteristics of physicians and administrators may result in conflicts if both parties fail to properly deal with each other (see chart on next page).

One way to reduce conflict between administrators and physicians is to clearly define the duties and responsibilities of physician managers and administrators. A common problem in medical groups is having the administrator and the medical director both thinking they are in charge.

"Coordination of the responsibilities of physician managers and the administrators is essential. Typically the responsibility of the physician manager is mainly to set goals, objectives, medical standards and group policies. The medical group administrator then focuses on operationally achieving the goals and objectives in accordance with standards and policies that are in force ... The problem most medical groups faced was that, although management power was held by the medical group administrator, the expectation was that the administrator would merely handle internal operations. The administrator's traditional job was not to be outward looking and in the lead of a changing marketplace."[18]

Ten common mistakes administrators make in dealing with physicians [17]

Mistake	Comments
1. Looking for an approach to physicians;	• There is no such thing as a single successful approach to physicians.
2. Cronyism;	• Favoritism usually generates a significant number of disenchanted outsiders.
3. Fear of physicians;	• Job security is a strong motivator.
4. Expecting loyalty;	• Many [administrators] believe they can buy a physician's loyalty.
5. Thinking that educating and involving physicians is a waste of time;	• [Administrators] have discovered that time spent developing the support of reasonable physicians is productive.
6. Being perceived as unavailable;	• When a physician calls an [administrator] he or she is told that the [administrator] is in a meeting.
7. Failing to put the monkey of adequate communication on the backs of physician leaders;	• A physician [leader] can be particularly effective in helping physicians establish communication.
8. Delegating physician matters to a junior executive or middle manager;	• Think of dealing with reasonable physicians as if they are senior executives of other companies.
9. Believing the health care business really is identical to other businesses; and	• The biggest difference between health care and commercial business is the presence of the practicing physician.
10. Being slow to establish the position of (physician) services.	• Physicians increasingly understand the disadvantages of having part-time leaders.

Physicians also make their share of mistakes in dealing with medical group administrators.

Eight common mistakes physicians make when dealing with administrators [19]

1. Refusal to recognize a higher authority;
2. Overgeneralizing;
3. Refusal to take time to understand and use key principles;
4. Believing that only practicing physicians understand the details of medical practice;
5. The George Steinbrenner mistake – "Things not going well, fire the manager";
6. Over resistance to change;
7. Thinking that the general public still loves and has confidence in the medical profession – as one physician said, "Once, we were on a pedestal. Now, I don't think we are anywhere near the museum"; and
8. Being arrogant.

There also is a difference in how physicians and administrators make decisions. In the hospital, if the CEO tells subordinates to do something, they do it. In the clinic, if the CEO tells one of the physicians to do something, he [she] may find himself [herself] in an argument. There is constant friction and a tug of war . . . [As one hospital CEO put it:] 'In the hospital it takes us longer to make a decision, but once we make it, we can hold it. Physicians in the clinic can make decisions faster, but they usually have trouble standing by the decision once it is made.'" [20]

The 'right' medical group physicians

The success of medical groups is dependent on the quality of their physician members. Many medical groups have a difficult time weeding "bad apple" physicians from their ranks. Problems may be overlooked until they get to a critical point, when the group faces possible lawsuits. Some medical groups require all group physicians to vote on the termination of a peer, which can make the termination process embarrassing to the affected party.

The 'right' medical group physicians

- committed to high quality and cost-effective care;
- meet professional competency standards;
- contribute to patient, staff and peer satisfaction;
- work collaboratively in a group setting;
- productive, yet efficient;
- willing to give up personal autonomy for the "good of the whole"; and
- willing to share their income, expenses and governance.

Medical groups should have appropriate credentialing standards that insure recruitment of high quality, cost-effective, group-minded physicians. Medical groups also should give physicians clear expectations of acceptable behaviors, develop incentives which reward the desired behaviors, and make physicians accountable (terminate them if necessary) when such behaviors are not followed.

Specialist-dominated multispecialty medical groups

Many multispecialty medical groups were formed by specialists to provide a primary care referral base for their practices. As these medical groups transition from fee-for-service care to capitated care, they usually experience difficulties in managing health care costs. Specialists may be reluctant to provide services at competitive rates or allocate capitation dollars to primary care physicians for "gatekeeper" functions.

Problems of specialist-dominated multispecialty medical groups

- Too high a ratio of specialists to primary care physicians to attract and retain managed care contracts
- Unwillingness of specialists to transfer income or capitation dollars to primary care physicians resulting in:
  - Non-competitive primary care physician compensation
  - Attrition of their primary care physician referral base
- Poor managed care performance from the high group cost structure

Physicians required by HMOs [21]

Total physicians required	Required by HMOs	1992 US M.D. supply	Percent over (under)
Physicians/100,000 members	129.25	180.1	39.3%
Percent of total physicians			
Primary care physicians	44.0%	36.5%	(17.2%)
Medical subspecialists	13.3%	18.0%	35.8%
Surgical specialists	33.8%	46.8%	38.7%
Hospital-based specialists	3.1%	4.2%	35.5%

As multispecialty medical groups transition to managed and capitated care, primary care physicians should be given the dominant role in medical group governance. This is difficult for some medical groups as primary care physicians may be less assertive than their specialist peers.

The 'worst possible guy' phenomenon

In group practices, it is common to assign certain areas of responsibility to certain physicians, either as individuals, committee chairmen or committee members. In many cases, it is "the worst possible guy (or gal)" who is chosen for assignment to specific areas of responsibility. Here are some actual examples:

Dr. Careful, as the newly elected chairman of the executive committee of the Awesome Medical Clinic was pondering on the problem of assigning chairmen to the 43 subcommittees in his 20-physician group. Thinking back on the twice-a-week, six-hour group meetings over the previous seven years, he recalled that Dr. Picky had frequently voiced concern over the quality of medical records. Frequently Dr. Picky's concerns related to an "i" not being dotted or a "t" crossed twice, but sometimes it was serious business like a change in the typeface on subsequent patient visits in the same chart.

Dr. Careful decided that it would be a good managerial strategy to appoint Dr. Picky chairman and sole member of the medical records committee. It would accomplish two very important objectives: (1) medical records would be in good hands, and (2) Dr. Picky would quit complaining at group meetings.

I think you already know how this turned out for the members of the Awesome Medical Clinic. Their records became perfect — flawless. But the expense of four more medical transcriptionists and all new typewriters with matching type style ate their lunch.

Another instance of the "worst possible guy" was the appointment of the most vocal complainer to the chair of the committee on accounts receivable, credit and collections. For some time, he had complained about his "good paying patients" being offended by delinquent account notices on their statements. Soon after he assumed his responsibilities as chairman of this important committee, the delinquent account notices disappeared from the statements and the complaints dropped off almost as much as the collection percentage. [22]

Just because someone talks a lot about something does not mean he or she should be in charge of it. Sometimes the loudest and most vocal critic is the worst choice to correct a problem.

Medical groups should assign responsibilities based on competence not interest (and more often to trained staff, not just part-time untrained physicians). As Walt Disney once said, "Whenever you're working on a project, always have one person who knows what he's doing."

Notes

[1]   "Corporate Culture, the Silent Governor," *Medical Group Management Journal*, May/June, 1989.

[2]   *The Physician Group Practice*, E. Jordan, p. 2.

[3]   *My Pulse Is Not What It Used to Be: The Leadership Challenges in Health Care*, Irwin M. Rubin, Ph.D. and C. Raymond Fernandez, M.D., p. 13.

[4]   *Integrated Health Care: Reorganizing the Physician, Hospital and Health Plan Relationship*, Coddington, Moore and Fischer, 1994, p. 126.

[5]   "Leadership Competencies for Physicians," *Healthcare Forum Journal*, July/August, 1993.

[6]   "Why Physicians Fail," *Physician Executive*, M. McCall and J. Clair, 1990, pp. 6-10.

[7]   Ibid., p. 9.

[8]   *Ambulatory Care Management and Practice*, Edited by A. Barnett, M.D. and G. Mayer, RN, EdD, FAAN, pp. 58-59.

9   "Leadership Competencies for Physicians," *Healthcare Forum Journal*, July/ August, 1993.

10 *Why Physicians in Group Practice Earn Less than Comparable Colleagues in Solo Practice*; a brief critical paper. Group Practice Management, Incorporated, Columbia, Mo., p. 2.

11 Ibid., p. 3.

12 *Ambulatory Care Management and Practice*, Edited by A. Barnett, M.D. and G. Mayer, RN, EdD, FAAN, pp. 56-57.

13 *The Physician Group Practice*, E. Jordan, pp. 143-144.

14 *Keys to Winning Physician Support*, by Richard Thompson, The American College of Physician Executives, 1991.

15 Ibid.

16 *My Pulse Is Not What It Used to Be: The Leadership Challenges in Health Care*, Irwin M. Rubin, Ph.D. and C. Raymond Fernandez, M.D., pp. 46-48.

17 *Keys to Winning Physician Support*, by Richard Thompson, The American College of Physician Executives, 1991.

18 *Ambulatory Care Management and Practice*, Edited by A. Barnett, M.D. and G. Mayer, R.N., Ed.D., FAAN, pp. 54, 56.

19 *Keys to Winning Physician Support*, by Richard Thompson, The American College of Physician Executives, 1991.

20 *Integrated Health Care: Reorganizing the Physician, Hospital and Health Plan Relationship*, Coddington, Moore and Fischer, 1994, pg. 125.

21 "Big Mergers in New England," *Integrated Healthcare Report*, Edited by John D. Cochrane, August, 1994, p. 9.

22 *Why Physicians in Group Practice Earn Less than Comparable Colleagues in Solo Practice*; a brief critical paper. Group Practice Management, Incorporated, Columbia, Mo., p. 2.

CHAPTER SIX

Medical Group Economics

Does bigger make better?

Most businesses enjoy economies of scale. The more units of a product or a service produced, generally the lower the per unit cost. Medical practices organized into groups appear in the aggregate to be the unhappy exception to the principle of economies of scale. In fact, the opposite seems to be true: the larger the medical group, the less efficient the operations. Of course, there are always exceptions to every rule.

1995 Medical Group Management Association Cost Survey (based 1992 Data) [1]

Medical group ratios	<11 M.D.s	11-25 M.D.s	26-50 M.D.s	51-75 M.D.s	76-150 M.D.s	150+ M.D.s
FTE support staff/ FTE M.D.s	4.52 FTEs	4.75 FTEs	4.94 FTEs	4.98 FTEs	5.24 FTEs	4.60 FTEs
Accounts receivable/ FTE M.D.	$86,785	$111,918	$117,601	$96,799	$121,198	$121,546
Accounts receivable ratio	2.59 months	3.18 months	3.59 months	3.45 months	3.55 months	3.94 months
Support staff salaries/ FTE M.D.	$92,485	$101,219	$103,760	$109,679	$121,771	$109,943
Total operating expenses/FTE M.D.	$210,794	$238,956	$253,647	$250,534	$279.433	$292,988
Margins available for provier distributions	43.08% of total revenue	46.72% of total revenue	46.05% of total revenue	45.13% of total revenue	45.39% of total revenue	45.82% of total revenue

This trend (increased overhead, longer collection periods and reduced margins available for physician distributions) only worsens as medical groups increase their percentage of managed care. "Groups relying most heavily on managed care employed 5.23 staff FTEs per physician in 1994, compared with only 4.75 staff per physician in groups without managed care." [2]

There is a danger in looking at these statistics to infer that large groups are unable to achieve true economies of scale. Logic dictates that, as duplicate staff and functions are eliminated, operations consolidated and leverage achieved through large scale purchasing and contracting, that efficiencies should result. In many large groups, other factors often offset benefits achieved through these economies of scale (bureaucratic red tape, inadequate or improper management, too many committees, mushrooming support staff, etc.). In addition, more staff and overhead per group physician are not necessarily bad; the extra resources may contribute additional revenues and compensation for these group physicians. However, because of ineffective medical group management, all too often spending extra results in fewer efficiencies and reduced group physician income. Like all statistics, this data needs more study to determine what it really means. Group Practice Management, Incorporated, says there is plenty of blame to go around for medical groups lacking economies of scale:

> Medical economists have observed this financial phenomenon with curiosity for years. Unfortunately they have traditionally allowed their curiosity to deteriorate to disinterest after being advised by physicians that it was all to blame on administrators, and in turn, advised by administrators that it was most certainly the fault of the group physicians, themselves. One might think that the accountants' efforts should have shed some light on this problem, but alas, these accountants are no more economists than administrators are physicians, nor vice versa on both counts. [3]

Medical groups must have the will and leadership to achieve true economies of scale. With centralization of services, support systems and staff comes a certain loss of physician autonomy and flexibility. Also "large" medical groups need to keep their entrepreneurial spirit, and not let bureaucracy get in the way of efficiency. Physician incentives for effective group performance are important factors in keeping medical group operations lean and mean.

The successful medical groups over the long-term will be those who are willing to invest in their future and not just the present. This may mean taking less physician income now to have more in the future.

Group practices without walls

Some physicians forming groups would like to have their cake and eat it too; keep the autonomy and decentralized operational structure of a solo practice and yet get the benefits of centralized management, contracting and support services (a typical "group practice without walls"). Since this usually results in no decrease in actual individual physician overhead, many "group practices without walls" do not work. They only add overhead to existing practice economics instead of saving money. In many cases, it is the health system which has agreed to create the "group practice without walls" that gets stuck footing the extra bills.

Gary Susnara, senior vice-president of Sutter Health Systems in Sacramento, Calif., describes the problems Sutter Health had with its development of an aligned "group practice without walls," the Sacramento Sierra Medical Group, Sacramento, Calif.:

> In my view, the medical group without walls is substantially flawed if you think you are developing a medical group, because you are not ... You basically put a corporate structure over the top of a bunch of independent practices. How will you pay for that corporate structure? You don't necessarily do away with the same day-to-day expenses you have in running individual practices. Yet you don't have the access to ancillary dollars ...
>
> So ultimately you are not generating the same amount of revenue that a traditional group practice does to pay for its overhead. You are just duplicating your overhead ...
>
> Effective managed care contracting requires tight organization and control. In a group practice without walls, you are spread all over a geographic region. Some doctors don't even know other doctors in the group.
>
> The model itself is flawed. It is the last way [for physicians] to dodge the bullet. The doctors can keep their independence [they may think]. "We will all make lots of money, and we won't be under the control of anybody." The fact of the matter is that it doesn't work that way and it is not going to work that way. If someone else wants to do it [build a group practice without walls], I wish them Godspeed. [4]

Coddington, Moore and Fischer list five reasons for the failure of the Sacramento Sierra Medical Group:

- Sac Sierra had too many practice sites — at one point, there were 70 locations. Many of these were clustered around the medical center so they did not provide geographic coverage.

- Because of the multiple locations, Sac Sierra was unable to realize significant revenues from centralizing ancillary services, such as laboratory and radiology. There were no economies of scale. In fact, because of the central administrative offices, overhead was higher than it would have been without the association.
- Primary care physicians' net incomes were falling. The organization lacked a funding source to prop up these incomes to be competitive with what other physicians were earning in the Sacramento marketplace.
- Sac Sierra failed to develop a corporate culture among participating physicians. Physicians continued to practice in their own office settings and had little reason to share their experiences with others in the group.
- Including specialists in the organization did not yield the additional hoped-for source of revenue to support primary care physicians. Specialists eventually left the group with the blessing of the primary care physicians and Sutter Health. [5]

Physicians joining medical groups must clearly understand the trade-offs between the loss of their individual autonomy and the increased efficiencies and physician incomes possible through achieving true group practice.

Incurred But Not Reported claims

Those medical groups who have agreed to accept capitated payments from health plans may suffer from inadequate accounting and cash reserves for Incurred But Not Reported (IBNR) claims. These claims arise when medical groups refer medical services to non-group providers for patients enrolled under the medical group capitated care plans (payment for such services being the responsibility of the medical group). Normally the extent and cost of such services are not predetermined and are billed to the medical group from these outside providers after services are rendered (usually on a discounted fee-for-service basis).

Medical groups may lack appropriate tracking systems to measure the appropriateness or amount of these outstanding claims. In addition, accounting personnel (and outside auditors) for some medical groups may even be unaware that these claims exist or need to be recorded, especially since several medical groups still use cash basis accounting.

Having capitation dollars "in the bank" may tempt administrators to use these available funds to maintain levels of physician compensation while paying IBNR out of future capitation revenues. That is like "borrowing from Peter to pay Paul."

Medical groups should put into place appropriate systems to track and properly reserve dollars for IBNR claims on a timely basis. Groups should adopt the accrual basis of accounting to better track their actual liabilities in a complex managed care world.

Sending out the business

It is sometimes very difficult to convince group physicians that they are "shooting themselves in the foot" when they send business out of the group. Group physicians may have all kinds of excuses: "I don't like Joe (group physician)," "Bill (group physician) never returns my calls," "Mary (non-group physician) is the best surgeon in town." Instead of trying to fix internal problems, it is sometimes easier for group physicians to send business elsewhere. Sometimes the medical group has real problems matching price or quality with outsiders. This frequently results in significant losses of potential group revenues and profits and higher group costs under capitated managed care programs. But it is usually very difficult for group administrators and physician leaders to get group physicians to correct this problem.

Group physicians should have a direct incentive for retaining group business. Systems should be in place to both track referrals outside the medical group as well as to insure proper feedback on problems between group physicians that limit internal referrals.

You want my outside income?

Some group physicians see nothing wrong with significant "moonlighting" activities outside the group, even if such activities interfere with their ability to dedicate their full time efforts to the medical group they work for. In addition, these physicians usually want this outside income to pass through to them without any deductions (assuming it is reported to and received by the medical group). Frequently such activities put these physicians in a part-time status, while the group remains responsible to pay full-freight for dedicated support personnel and office space.

An additional related concern is investments by group physicians in ventures which compete directly with the group. Many medical groups prohibit such investments in their physician employment contracts. Some physicians try to avoid these restrictions by having spouses make their outside investments for them.

Medical groups should have clear, enforced policies prohibiting competitive outside investments of time and money by their physicians (and physicians' spouses) to support group cohesion and good economics.

Lessors vs. lessees

When only some of the group physicians own group medical office buildings or major pieces of group equipment leased to the medical group, the group is headed for trouble. This conflict of interest between physician lessors and lessees has caused several groups to split up. It also becomes a problem when retiring or terminating physicians keep their ownership interests in group facilities and equipment after leaving the group. The lessor physicians may want as high a rent as possible and frequently build in "appreciation clauses" to reward themselves while the lessee physicians want the lowest possible rent. If the lessor physicians are in a majority control position within a medical group, high medical group overhead is usually the result.

Groups who wish to avoid the lessor/lessee problem mandate that ALL or NO group physicians be allocated an equal ownership position in group assets, and require that retiring and terminating physicians dispose of any group ownership interests.

Lack of sharing of group income

Those multispecialty groups (or primary care groups integrated with health systems) that do not recognize the need for paying primary care physicians competitively risk losing these physicians to other groups or systems that recognize their importance in managing patient care. Several methods exist to share medical group income with primary care physicians. They include group compensation plans, profit-sharing plans and capitation allocation plans. Without such sharing of income many primary care physicians would not make as much in a multispecialty group practice as they would in solo practice (for all the reasons above and below). Sharing medical group income with primary care physicians also has a downside: many primary care physicians in multispecialty medical groups are perceived to be "lazier" than their solo practice peers. Because of group income sharing, they may not have to work as hard to make an equivalent income.

Multispecialty groups (and integrated health systems) need to recognize the need to share medical group income with primary care physicians for group (and integrated health system) success. Compensation systems should be designed to provide competitive market-based compensation to all physicians.

Group growth problems

Several medical groups allow individual physician members to determine when additional physicians should be recruited to meet patient and payer demands. Since most groups still pay physicians based on individual physician revenues generated, established physician members may block the group from recruiting a new physician until they are servicing at least two practices so that they will not experience a pay cut during the first year the new physician comes. This causes two problems: (1) patients are faced with long wait times trying to get into the established physician's practice until the new recruit comes, and (2) generally there is a long lag time between the time of the decision by this established physician to recruit and the ability of the group to sign a new recruit. By this time, patients may become so dissatisfied with group service that they go elsewhere, leaving the new physician recruit without enough to do upon arrival. This could result in the new physician recruit leaving as well.

Another major problem with group growth can be accounts receivable. New physicians expect a salary from day one. But groups still having partial or full fee-for-service practices have time lags between the date new physicians bill for services rendered and the date the group collects. Some groups deal with this problem by "lending salaries" to new physicians. They are recovered over a short period through lower compensation to these new physicians. This loan process can strain groups going through major growth spurts, as established group physicians may have to "kick in" significant portions of their own incomes to help get new physicians up and running.

Groups that do not grow ultimately die. It is critical that medical groups control recruiting at the board level in accordance with a recruitment plan tied to the group's strategic and financial plans, rather than at the individual physician or specialty department level. Medical groups should develop capital to fund growth (with a capital partner and/or internally generated reserves).

Physician buy ins and buy outs

Many medical groups are caught in a continual Ponzi Scheme: they have to recruit new physicians who will "buy into" the group to "buy out" physicians who retire, terminate group employment or pass away. Since medical groups do not normally have enough cash to buy out leaving physicians (groups generally have no cash, only accounts receivable and some tangible assets), these groups usually have to sign notes for large amounts to fund these buy outs over a period of time. New physician recruits can provide cash for these buy outs as they buy in. Large buy ins are becoming a major deterrent for medical groups in recruiting new physicians.

If new physicians are not recruited to replace leaving physicians, the medical group with leaving physicians frequently has no option other than leveraging or selling group assets to provide buy out capital. Most groups cannot easily partially or fully liquidate their assets. This gives physicians with equity a "hammer" that can destroy a group if significant numbers of physicians leave at one time.

Many medical groups have used various methods to get around the buy in and buy out problems. Some groups have "cashed out" their equity physicians by selling their assets to a hospital or other capital partner, or have formed medical foundations. New medical groups should be structured to minimize or eliminate buy in and buy out requirements.

Accumulation of medical group reserves

Medical groups organized as professional corporations usually distribute all cash at the end of the tax year to avoid double taxation (at the corporate and individual physician shareholder level). This results in these medical groups historically being "cash poor," with reserves primarily represented by two assets: accounts receivable and any tangible assets held (facilities and equipment). Since these two assets usually are owned by group shareholder physicians, in some groups these assets cannot be leveraged to meet group capital needs.

It's difficult for medical groups to agree to reduce current physician income to provide future reserves for group needs. Some group physicians mistrust their own governance to look after their own long-term interests. They demand either current dollars or vested retirement plan dollars, leaving no reserves for future group needs. In addition, should group capital needs arise, these same physicians usually are reluctant to invest personal capital for group investment needs. However, some physicians are willing to make large personal investments outside the group, sometimes in competitive joint ventures or investments their brother-in-law stockbroker recommended, with little or no due diligence or oversight.

If medical groups do not accumulate reserves, they will be unable to grow and prosper. More and more often today, medical groups are being forced to align with a capital partner to survive.

Evidence of sufficient medical group reserves

- solid cash position;
- adequate capital base to support growth;
- low debt-to-equity ratio;
  good debt service coverage ratio;
- efficient, well-managed and capitalized operations;
- proper accrual of liabilities; and
- market-based competitive compensation of physicians.

Medical groups today have several alternatives to avoid the taxation problems of professional corporations while building adequate working capital reserves. These alternatives include forming a medical foundation, integrating with a nonprofit tax-exempt health system, and aligning with another capital partner.

Annual budgets and long-range plans

For years, many medical groups operated without annual budgets or long-range plans. With the increased need for capital and the increased complexity of the managed health care environment, groups are now faced with developing financial and strategic plans for the first time.

It is absolutely critical that medical groups operate from annual budgets and long-range strategic and financial business plans. The days of raising rates to cover costs are long over. Medical groups should allocate group resources for financial and strategic planning advice. All strategic and financial plans should be tracked against medical group goals and objectives.

Notes

[1] Cost Survey: 1995 Report Based on 1994 Data, Medical Group Management Association, 1995, pp. 70-87..

[2] Ibid., p. 95.

[3] *Why Physicians in Group Practice Earn Less than Comparable Colleagues in Solo Practice*; a brief critical paper. Group Practice Management, Incorporated, Columbia, Mo., p.1.

[4] "Prototype Group Practice Without Walls Reveals Cracks," *Medical Staff Strategy Report*, September, 1993.

[5] *Integrated Health Care: Reorganizing the Physician, Hospital and Health Plan Relationship*, Coddington, Moore and Fischer, 1994, p. 40.

Physician compensation and benefits

Symptoms of a failing compensation plan

Susan Cejka, of Cejka and Company in St. Louis, Mo., describes various symptoms of a failing medical group compensation plan:

Symptoms of a failing compensation plan [1]

Issues	Possible areas of concern
• The practice continually needs to borrow to cover operating deficits • Physician turnover is increasing. • Unable to recruit the quality and quantity of physicians needed to meet demand. • Arguments among physicians are frequent and heated. • Overhead appears to be uncontrollable. • Physicians have become apathetic and do not take part in clinic meetings and decisions. • There is increasing pressure on the administrator to craft special deals.	• There is a fixed payout percentage. • There is no cost accounting for compensation or management of resource utilization. • A production-based formula is used in a fixed revenue environment. • Plan is not current with payment sources. • Compensation is not competitive. • The pay plan discriminates against particular specialists. • Culture is undermined by the pay plan. • Compensation is not competitive. • The plan is complex and not easily understood. • Unclear link exists between effort and compensation. • Group goals unclear. • Biases and subsidies have resulted in physicians exploiting the system. • There are hidden subsidies. • There is no accountability for costs. • There are too many special deals. • Growth is uncontrolled. • The plan is not clearly understood. • The plan is not perceived to be fair. • Specific deals are made outside context of the plan. • The plan is not fair. • Unclear group goals.

However, Cejka indicates there is no perfect compensation plan.

> Before sorting out the issues, it should be understood that there is no perfect compensation plan. All plans, no matter how carefully crafted, include biases that favor one physician or specialty ... The key to developing a successful compensation plan is to understand how the biases ... impact physicians and group practice competitiveness and to ensure ... the achievement of long-term goals ...
>
> Compensation plans are not static documents. Changes in the marketplace, technology, and group size and mix all generate a need to review and revise the compensation plan ... A successful group makes frequent although incremental changes to the compensation plan to reflect changes in its strategic plan and the health care environment.
>
> The compensation plan must be easily understood ... The compensation plan is meant to motivate behavior. If the plan is so complex that few can understand [it], then there is little chance that the plan will have this effect ... Physicians exhibit great concern over the way the pie is split. More often, the problem is the size of the pie ...
>
> The ability of the group to achieve long-range goals and objectives is inextricably linked to the structure and content of the compensation plans ... The compensation plan can motivate physicians to work toward the common goals of the group, modify physician behavior with regard to practice style and efficiency, and increase communication flow among the specialties. A compensation plan can build group culture, but, more realistically, it can shape or influence group culture ...
>
> The plan itself cannot be expected to be a substitute for strong group leadership ... It does not replace culture, values or morals, although it may affect them ... It does not replace long-range planning or the institutional mission. The plan cannot make everyone equal; it cannot erase inequities between specialties that have existed for many years. Finally, the compensation plan will not cause or cure a serious case of terminal greed.[2]

Cejka's analysis is only a partial list of the problems medical groups experience with physician compensation plans (see below for more). There is certainly no more controversial aspect of group practice than physician compensation plans.

In this time of dynamic change in health care, compensation plans need to evolve in response to market forces. Medical groups need to design flexible and adaptable compensation plans to meet their goals and objectives as well as provide appropriate incentives for desired physician behaviors. There is a saying among medical group administrators: "There are three medical group compensation plans: this year's, last year's and next year's."

Spending money you don't have

Many group practice administrators frequently are faced with a difficult decision: the financial results for the year just ended do not match with the prior year's, but the group physicians expect to be paid just as much (or more) as they were last year. This problem is becoming a reality as medical groups face escalating costs along with declining reimbursements.

Frequently, medical groups pay flat monthly salaries to their physicians and then adjust at the end of each quarter or the end of the year. Since some groups are not willing to invest the money required for good internal accounting systems and staff, physicians may not become aware of necessary pay adjustments or shortfalls until after the end of the year. This causes real problems when the year-end adjustment results in group physicians being overpaid. Administrators have limited choices when this happens: come clean and tell the truth to the physicians (and get the physicians to pay back their overpayments immediately or over time) or borrow to pay group physicians based on their expectations (and adjust against their next year's income). The latter strategy has been the death spiral for some groups, who usually never face the music, but continue to leverage assets to satisfy physician demands.

These medical group administrators are caught in a "Catch-22": if they do not satisfy their physicians, the affected physicians will threaten to leave, fire the administrator, etc. (related to the administrator insecurity problem above). If they satisfy the physicians they will be strapped with additional debt without means of servicing it properly.

Medical group administrators need to be honest and say when there will be insufficient funds with which to pay expected physician compensation. In addition, medical groups need monthly and quarterly reporting mechanisms to group physicians so that there will be no year-end surprises.

Confuse 'em or lose 'em

Some group administrators get physicians to cooperate with pay changes by designing profit distribution formulas that are so complicated physicians do not know whether their pay went up or down. According to Cejka: "Complexity is frequently related to weak group leadership, the absence of a strategic plan, conflicting long-term goals and cultural bias toward making special deals as a way of placating the most vocal members of the group."[3] Using a complex formula can have physicians so confused, they do not know what happened to them. For example, an administrator might say: "Your percentage of net billable dollars went up, but your percentage of capitated revenues went down, etc."

Physician compensation plans should be easy to understand and implement. Administrators can help facilitate better communication regarding physician compensation by getting group physician leaders to help deliver the message using a physician-run "physician compensation committee."

The deferred bonus approach

Some administrators get around the year-end pay adjustment or bonus shortfall problem by deferring bonuses until sufficient cash flow is generated in the next fiscal year to pay last year's expected bonuses. This deferral may result in group physicians, whose expectation was a large bonus on X date, learn that neither the amount of the bonus nor the expected timing of the bonus distribution is realized — sometimes after the responsible administrator is long gone.

The successful medical group administrator provides frequent, timely and accurate updates to group physicians on financial trends, and does not use future receipts to pay current physician compensation.

Measuring physician work effort/contributions

As professionals, physicians usually resent having time reports or other mechanisms to measure their work effort. Most medical groups measure physician productivity by accounting for professional revenues on an individual and aggregate physician basis. Some groups also track physician hours based on automated scheduling systems. Unfortunately, neither system adequately measures "physician group contributions." Some physicians have learned how to upcode fees to increase their professional revenues, and they may or may not efficiently and satisfactorily provide productive and appropriate patient care for the hours they work. Depending on incentives for physician productivity, physicians also may work the system to see only patients who pay well. They may avoid patients who are on low-pay plans or who take more time to process (Medicare, etc.).

Successful medical groups are developing physician evaluation processes which reward other factors besides billings or hours worked. These discretionary income systems are being used by several large medical groups as a supplement to guaranteed base salaries for their physicians.

Nonproductive physicians

There are some physicians who, no matter what incentives are incorporated in compensation systems, are unable to be productive. They may have a practice style that makes productivity impossible (slow in processing paperwork, talk to patients endlessly, never show up on time, afraid to bill for time spent because of the fear of losing patients, etc.). They may be so unpopular with patients that they can not maintain a full practice. In addition, some physicians just do not want to work very hard, are not very entrepreneurial or work in a group primarily for security reasons.

Sometimes groups face the problem of a nonproductive physician when an older physician starts to slow down (such as an OB-Gyn physician who wants to give up obstetrics, or a surgeon who wants to concentrate on an office practice, etc.). Frequently, this physician feels entitled to the same perks enjoyed by full-time group physicians (e.g., the same overhead percentage as the group, even though his or her overhead percentage has increased because of the need to cover fixed costs for a full-time practice with only part-time practice revenues). After all, "The physician has paid his or her dues."

Groups need to recognize when they have problems with nonproductive physicians. They should take appropriate actions in their compensation plans to adjust nonproductive physician compensation and overhead allocations accordingly. Having policies or plans laid out in advance regarding pending retirement also can be advantageous (developing a slide on compensation that is applicable to all physicians as of a certain age).

Transitioning from fee-for-service to capitation

Medical groups with capitated revenues must face the challenge of redesigning physician compensation systems from fee-for-service incentives if they wish to properly provide incentives to physicians for capitated patient care(in which revenues are based on a flat amount per enrollee regardless of medical services rendered). Groups partially capitated and partially fee-for-service have to deal with schizophrenic tendencies of their physicians who believe they need to do more for fee-for-service patients and less for capitated patients. Those groups getting into capitation which continue their fee-for-service incentive systems for a period of time usually have significant difficulties controlling their managed care costs. Physicians and medical groups expect large increases in the percentage of their practices that will be capitated in the next few years: One recent survey by John Alden, a Miami insurance company, showed that physicians accepting per-person [capitated] contracts expect such patients to provide about two-thirds of their income in five years, compared with 16 percent now. [4]

Various compensation systems exist to pay physicians differently for capitated care; however, the best systems provide incentives for physicians to provide the same cost-effective, quality care (not more, not less) for all patients. John McDonald, administrator of the Mulliken Medical Group in Southern California, described the issues of changing incentives in this way: "Groups must modify physician compensation and scrap production-based systems. Compensation must be tied to quality, not to any type of system in which the individual can control the supply side of the equation, as in the fee-for-service system."[5] Mulliken Medical Group compensates its physicians from three sources:

- From practice: Physicians are compensated for the amount of time they spend seeing patients and providing quality care in a cost-effective manner.
- From management: Physicians in administration are compensated for management responsibilities.
- From capital: Physicians have a right to return on investment for capital invested in the business, equipment and facilities.[6]

Medical groups that hang on to productivity-based formulas too long are headed for trouble as they transition to capitated care. Medical groups need to design their compensation systems to reward the appropriate physician behaviors required in a new managed care world.

Compensation formulas for capitated care should reward physician efficiency as well as quality of care and patient service. Just "capitating" physicians can result in patient dumping, underutilization, patient dissatisfaction, and a myriad of other problems.

Coupling capitation with bonus systems that measure and reward physician performance provides a means to ensure patients are well cared for in an efficient and effective manner.

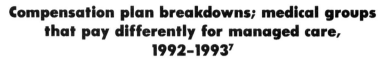

Compensation plan breakdowns; medical groups that pay differently for managed care, 1992-1993[7]

1993   1992

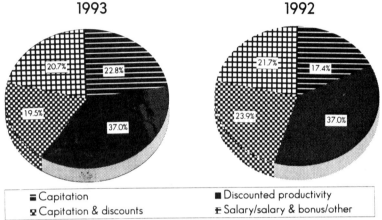

≡ Capitation	■ Discounted productivity
⚯ Capitation & discounts	⌶ Salary/salary & bonus/other

Individual vs. group cost accounting

To be fair in compensating group physicians, some medical groups go through convoluted cost accounting formulas to properly allocate costs by department and/or individual physician. While this helps make physicians accountable for the costs of their operations, it also adds administrative costs and makes "group-think" difficult: "I don't want to spend group dollars for THAT because it might add $___ to my individual cost allocation." On the other hand, groups that have no individual physician accountability for group costs run the risk of having group physicians wanting to buy everything "since the 'group' is paying for it."

The best approach to individual vs. group cost accounting is probably a mixture of individual physician accountability and group accountability for medical group expenditures.

The 'sacred formula'

Medical group compensation formulas are certainly not static, but do seem to take on a sacred status while in place within medical groups. In some groups, if there is any deviance from the agreed-upon formula, the entire medical group needs to meet and agree with the change. This frequently hamstrings medical group administrators who have to open a major debate among group physicians whenever minor adjustments are required (to retain a key group physician, for example). This open debate process can cause major internal friction between physicians and often results in more harm than good.

Another problem with formulas is that they may not reflect actual market conditions. Since they are usually based on arbitrary mathematical algorithms, they usually cannot deal with changing market dynamics. This can result in individual group physicians being paid over or under the local market which ultimately will result in only the "underpaid" physicians leaving the group.

Some administrators have avoided the group discord that occurs with "full disclosure" of compensation formulas by using the secret approach. This is when all physician compensation decisions and discussions are only held one-on-one between the administrator and the physician affected. (Individual physician compensation information may be kept under lock and key.) In these groups, physicians know they are not to discuss their individual compensation with their colleagues.

Medical groups need to have their management and governance structures responsible for administering and modifying physician compensation plans. If every compensation plan change requires all group physicians to voice their opinions, group disunity and discord (and physician attrition) probably will result.

Physician vs. patient satisfaction

A tension that permeates many medical groups is whether physician or patient satisfaction has first priority. This is especially true if physicians are compensated solely on productivity (billings or hours worked) and satisfying patients is not an incentive (the norm for most medical groups). Unfortunately, some medical groups may subconsciously give priority to physician satisfaction over patient satisfaction.

Medical groups need to develop measurement systems that track patient satisfaction and reward physician behaviors accordingly. Compensating physicians on only productivity incentives may negatively affect patient satisfaction.

"If you want to have great customer relationships, you never focus on the customer — you always focus on what gave you great customer service — the employees who provide service."
—Walt Disney

What's more important?

Satisfying physicians	Satisfying patients
• increased incomes	• reduced health care costs
• high capitation rates	• low premium rates
• restricted physician access	• open physician access
• few locations	• several locations
• low overhead	• increased service
• flexible scheduling	• set appointments
• daytime hours	• extended hours
• over booking/long patient waits	• short wait times

Retirement plans

Physicians have notorious reputations for being bad investors. Group Practice Management, Incorporated, describes problems medical groups often have with their retirement plans:

Medical group problems with retirement plans [8]

- too much cash-value type of insurance in the retirement plans;
- tax-shelter type investments in the retirement plans;
- a buy and hold philosophy of equity investing;
- heavy real estate investments in the retirement plans; and
- excessive costs in the form of commissions, fees and other charges.

As described by Group Practice Management, Incorporated, medical groups often "buy high" and "sell low" when investing in their retirement plans:

> After many years of analyzing the investment results of different medical groups retirement funds, we have identified a consistent pattern and we have labeled it, "buy-high, sell-low" ... it is a very serious drain on assets which were intended for retirement of the members of the group ...
>
> The retirement funds of a medical group are usually under the control of a small number of physicians ... They are responsible to different people of different ages with wide differences in needs and wants ... they are "under the gun" for short-term performance and long-term performance ...

After observing the incompetence of their selected advisor for a period of time, [they] are likely to dismiss him [her] in favor of a newly-found investment star ... Advisor #1 had purchased these investments and then they went down in price (that's why he [she] got dismissed), and now our new hero must sell them to correct the mistakes of his predecessor. And the [physicians] have indirectly bought high and sold low. [9]

Most medical groups would do well to invest their retirement plans in a diversified group of no-load mutual funds and stay out of the "investing" business. Most physicians should concentrate on practicing medicine, and let professional investors manage their money, using long-term strategies and balanced funds.

Notes

[1] *Ambulatory Care Management and Practice*, Edited by A. Barnett, M.D. and G. Mayer, RN, EdD, FAAN, p. 80.

[2] Ibid., p. 75-76.

[3] Ibid., p. 77.

[4] "Health Plans Force Change In the Way Doctors Are Paid,' *The New York Times*, Feb. 9. 1995.

[5] *Integrated Health Care: Reorganizing the Physician, Hospital and Health Plan Relationship*, Coddington, Moore and Fischer, 1994, p. 109.

[6] Ibid., p. 77.

[7] *Physician Compensation and Production Survey: 1994 Report Based on 1993 Data*, Medical Group Management Association, 1994, p. 16.

[8] *Ambulatory Care Management and Practice*, Edited by A. Barnett, M.D. and G. Mayer, RN, EdD, FAAN, p. 26.

[9] *Why Physicians in Group Practice Earn Less than Comparable Colleagues in Solo Practice:* a brief critical paper, Group Practice Management, Incorporated, Columbia, Mo., p. 26.

C H A P T E R   E I G H T

Medical Group Operations

Medical records always are a problem

Almost without exception, the larger the medical group, the greater the problems with medical records:

Medical group problems with medical records

- Physicians sneak records out of the medical group to catch up at home, then leave the charts in the trunk of their car, in their briefcase, in their study at home or at their summer cabin. When asked where the patient charts are, they may forget or claim they do not know.
- Several physicians want access to a single chart simultaneously (e.g., the primary care physician, the orthopedist and the neurosurgeon). Since there are not duplicate or computerized charts, one of the physicians hides the chart in his/her office so that he/she is guaranteed access to it.
- Verbal battles occur between nursing personnel, reception personnel and chartroom personnel. The text contains the phrases, "I gave you that chart!" and "No, you didn't."
- Some medical records are kept at a central location with satellite offices only having partial medical records (select copies) because of the difficulty in transferring record data via fax or courier.
- Physicians want all charts available when they want them, but cannot understand why the overhead for chartroom personnel is so high.
- Physicians keep charts in their offices until they get time to process dictation, write histories or do billing. This results in conflicts between physicians and chartroom personnel who need to get the chart to another physician for a patient visit.
- Loose papers, such as lab results, pile up in wild confusion in the chartroom because no one has time to pull all the relevant charts to file the loose papers.

(continued on next page)

Medical group problems with medical records
(continued)

- Physicians and personnel claim: "I am sorry, but the chart must be lost." This can result in patients being seen without a medical chart – a significant liability risk.
- Various physicians refuse to follow group protocols regarding chart documentation. Some physicians may have illegible notes, lack of certain forms filled out or stacks of charts waiting for dictation.
- Some groups do not have systems that correlate appointments kept, chart pulls and billings. This can result in patients being seen without appropriate billings. One group had a computer report called the Missing Charges Report, but it was ignored because it tied missed billings to appointments made, not appointments kept. So many appointments were being canceled the report was meaningless.

Institute of Medicine and U.S. General Accounting Office records statistics [1]

- Physicians don't have access to patient medical records for more than 30 percent of visits.
- More than 11 percent of lab tests have to be redone because the results are not in the patient's record.
- Physicians spend 38 percent of their time handwriting notes in patient charts.

Many of the problems medical groups have with medical records would be solved if they invested in development of a computerized patient record (CPR).

> The CPR is an essential technology whose widespread adoption will catalyze major changes in physician practices. By moving the state-of-the-art in clinical data collection and access forward, the CPR stands to (i) improve patient care since effective access to patient records enhances the physician's ability to practice high quality, cost-effective medicine, (ii) reduce health care costs since physicians will gain access to usable clinical data necessary to manage costs and quality, and (iii) improve quality measurements since medical records data are fundamental to assessing physician practice patterns and patient outcomes ... Over the next five years, most physician practice organizations will implement many new systems along a migration path to the CPR ... [2]

To eliminate medical record problems, medical groups need to develop computerized medical records systems so that multiple parties can access the same records simultaneously. This requires a major capital investment which may require a capital partner.

Don't take my nurse away

Medical group physicians often think that group overhead is too high and that administration needs to cut nonphysician staff. These same physicians usually are reluctant to believe that the patient care staffing in their area (especially their own nurse) may be part of the problem. One of the difficult transitions groups have is changing from a one-nurse-to-every-doctor ratio to a nursing pool approach. In addition, if the medical group has a high ratio of registered nurses (RNs), it is very difficult to get supervising physicians to change the mix of nursing staff to a greater percentage of non-RNs.

One medical group voted on a major restructuring of its nursing staff. When its administration attempted to implement the restructuring (establishing a nursing pool, minor changes of the RN to non-RN mix, etc.), individual physicians went into an uproar. This resulted in the medical group board (all physicians) agreeing to table the restructuring.

Medical groups and medical group boards need to allow their administrators to manage staff while they practice medicine and set policy at the medical group board level.

My priority is more important

Administrators in groups owned and run by physicians have a difficult time balancing the demands of individual group physicians, each who may have their own pet projects and priorities. These individual group physicians may lobby their peers on the medical group board for special treatment. As a result, unbudgeted expenditures may get funding on an "immediate priority" basis, leaving budgeted expenditures without means of payment. It gets complicated for group administrators when individual physicians have conflicting agendas that need addressing simultaneously.

Strategic and financial plans and appropriate medical group governance should be in place and be followed in medical groups or anarchy may result.

Management information systems

More groups have probably gone under in the midst of a computer conversion than any other cause. Many times, these computer conversions result in delayed billings for several months and serious problems in lost data. One group in Northern California committed a cardinal sin which soon resulted in the group filing for bankruptcy: they went through a computer conversion in the midst of a major building project (along with other projects). Patients could not find parking spaces and were not sent bills for months — a recipe for disaster.

Effective management information systems

- data collected and reported on a timely and accurate basis;
- full spectrum of MIS systems offered:
  - managed care;
  - operations; and
  - links to outside systems;
- integrated, transparent systems; and
- properly staffed and supported central services.

Three physician practice management information systems product subgroups are emerging ... and will represent the majority of future growth in the market:

1. **managed care/decision support applications**, principally managed care administration, cost accounting and utilization management;
2. **electronic data interchange**, for transmitting electronic claims, tracking reporting requirements and sharing data, such as clinical graphics, medical images, pharmacy and laboratory information with trading partners; and
3. **computer-based patient record applications**, principally graphical user interfaces, clinical data repositories, knowledge-based systems and pen-based and voice recognition input devices. [3]

Medical groups need to carefully plan and implement computer conversions to avoid disrupting billings and operations. In addition, other projects should be delayed while computer conversions are in process.

Medical groups also need to allocate sufficient resources to develop effective, comprehensive management information systems that report timely and accurate data and are operated by competent support staff.

Hiring a physician's spouse

Medical groups are not immune to the same problems that other small businesses have when an owner's (physician's) spouse is employed in the business (medical group). In addition to the difficulty group administrators have in compensating and managing physician spouses, it is next to impossible to fire an incompetent one. These physician spouses can cause serious employee morale problems when they are not kept to the same standards as other employees, are paid more for equivalent work or are not disciplined appropriately. Just as bad are the problems that arise when a group physician gets romantically involved with an employee of the medical group, and that employee suddenly becomes exempt from accountability for performance.

Medical groups should adopt nepotism policies that prohibit employment of physician spouses and relatives to avoid potential personnel problems.

Appointment scheduling

Appointment scheduling is likely also to be a source of frustration in group management:

Areas of concern in appointment scheduling

- When physicians cancel patient appointments it is the patients and group staff who suffer – many physicians are so booked that the next available appointment may be six months out. However, when patients cancel appointments or are no-shows, most physicians want some compensation, such as a cancellation fee. This double standard becomes very apparent to group patients who may change physicians or leave the group.
- Some physicians in medical groups are always late. Rather than scheduling patients for when they are actually coming in, they schedule them a half-hour or hour before. This results in a continual backlog of dissatisfied patients waiting to be seen. Staff who attempt to bring sanity to this process by scheduling patients when the physician is actually available may be strongly lectured, disciplined or fired by the tardy physician.

(continued on next page)

Areas of concern in appointment scheduling
(continued)

- A common phenomenon in medical groups is the practice of over-booking patients. Physicians who want to maximize their practice income will overload their schedule (just as the airlines do) to insure that if there are no-shows, they will keep busy (and well-paid). Unfortunately, this usually results in lengthy patient wait times, patient dissatisfaction and patient attrition from the group. It also may result in a lack of new physician recruitment, even with increased patient demand.
- For physicians in groups paid based on gross charges, there may be no disincentive to see patients with poor credit histories or low reimbursements (Medicaid, etc.). Many medical group appointment systems have mechanisms to identify these patients, but usually require the physician be the final arbiter of whether the patient is seen. This may result in some physicians having large practices with "dead beats," with disproportionate writeoffs being absorbed by the group instead of the physician involved.

Enhanced appointment scheduling functions [4]

- Immediate notification of the medical records department when an appointment is made for today or tomorrow. This provides as much time as possible to locate and deliver the patient's medical record to the physician before the appointment time. This is especially critical when multiple physician offices and multiple chartrooms are involved, requiring the transportation of charts between offices.
- Automatic generation of visit slips with charge codes or descriptions tailored to the individual physician. Printing may be delayed until the patient arrives to conserve visit slips.
- Automatic search for the next available appointment based on a requested physician, specialty, office location, day of the week or time of day.
- Twenty-four-hour scheduling for departments with multiple shifts or around-the-clock coverage.
- Multiple appointment coordination when additional physician, room or equipment dependencies exist.
- On-line help to provide immediate field values and instruction.
- Interfaces with existing patient registration, HMO eligibility, HMO coverage and other related data bases.

The key to effective appointment scheduling is excellent computerized appointment scheduling systems, coupled with strong medical group governance and enforced appointment scheduling policies and procedures.

Billing for services rendered

While billing for services rendered is becoming less important as medical groups transition to capitation, it still accounts for the majority of most medical group revenue streams. Medical groups seem to share several common problems with billing for services rendered:

Medical group problems with billing for services rendered

- Medical groups may have physicians who are chronic "no-chargers" or "low-chargers." There may be several reasons for these physicians not charging or undercharging. These include group writeoffs of bad debts against the entire group instead of individual physicians, and insecurity of these physicians in potentially losing patients through charging high fees.
- Fee discounts to medical group patients may be out-of-control. As described by Group Practice Management, Incorporated in its publication, *Why Physicians in Group Practice Earn Less than Comparable Colleagues in Solo Practice,* "any one physician might have five discount situations; 10 doctors might have 50 discount arrangements ... Dr. A is Catholic so all priests, nuns, bishops, etc. receive discounts ... And of course we all want to discount nurses, lab techs ... It gets so bad that the receptionists not only won't accept cash anymore, but they are insisting that patients prove why they <u>aren't</u> entitled to a discount."
- Physicians are improperly coding fees for procedures resulting in potential penalties from Medicare and under- or over-billing of patients. These physicians may not be trained in proper coding techniques.
- Fee cards may be lost without followup to insure proper patient billing.

Medical groups should use effective computerized systems to monitor and enforce medical group policies regarding appropriate billing practices. Discounting, no-charging and low-charging should be minimized. As well, training programs should be offered to group physician and nonphysician staff on proper billing procedures.

Credit and collections

Medical groups may have easy extension of credit for services rendered. In addition to medical groups wanting to keep patient goodwill, several other factors contribute to medical groups being lenient in their credit policies.

Factors contributing to lenient medical group credit policies

- If medical group physicians are paid based on gross billings, they are provided incentives to see patients even if they are credit risks (especially if bad debts are allocated to the entire group and not to individual physicians).
- Some medical groups actually discourage payment at the time of service (by credit card, check or cash) because they have no procedure to calculate the amount of the bill. This contributes to services being rendered which may end up in collection.
- Medical groups may lack automated systems that screen patients prior to physician appointments.
- If medical group physicians are afraid of losing their patient base and not keeping busy, they may allow credit risk patients to be seen.

Group Practice Management, Incorporated, indicates that some medical groups lack effective controls and management in their credit and collection departments. They describe how some medical group credit and collection departments process accounts receivable:

> In many groups, collection people are given a thick alphabetical listing of delinquent accounts to work. In large groups, they only get the A's, B's and C's; in smaller groups, they get A through L or the whole alphabet.
>
> Anyway, they start out working every month on the A's — and they spend a lot of time on $10 and less accounts, but they never get back each month to the $500 delinquent balances at the end of their alphabetical section. [5]

Medical groups should establish credit and collection policies, then let administrative staff carry them out without physician interference. Credit and collection systems should be designed to get the most bang for the buck.

Managed care cost controls

It is difficult for physicians who have practiced in a fee-for-service environment to adapt to working under a managed and capitated care system. It takes significant capital as well as strong medical leadership to make a smooth transition. Frequently, medical groups experience poor managed care performance because of their inability to implement appropriate cost controls.

Problems with medical group managed care cost controls

- inadequate managed care information systems and procedures to report on and manage costs;
- medical group physician resistance to referral and utilization authorizations;
- retention of incentives that reward physicians for doing more rather than doing less;
- lack of direct physician incentives for controlling hospital costs and outside referrals;
- use of preferred expensive outside referral sources, instead of competitive (low cost, high quality) options;
- spotty and selective utilization review of only certain physicians (e.g., "Can't go after Ted, everyone likes him");
- payment of outside referral services using fee-for-service incentives rather than flat rates or subcapitation; and
- lack of control over drug costs or out-of-area costs (since they are covered by the health plan).

Elements of an effective managed care information system

- inpatient and outpatient utilization statistics;
- patient tracking – hospital, skilled nursing facilities, outpatient surgery, emergency room, etc.;
- monitoring of outside specialist referrals and authorizations;
- claims processing of referrals;
- insurance eligibility verification;
- comparison of hospital utilization costs to budget; and
- encounter data reporting to health plans.

Medical groups should invest in comprehensive, effective managed care information systems, and establish and follow well-organized managed care cost control procedures. Physician incentives should be aligned with managed care incentives, and utilization (inside and outside the group) should be appropriately monitored and controlled.

Measurement of effective performance

Medical groups have a difficult time measuring success. Medical group physicians may define it as more compensation than last year, group patients as lower prices or better service, and group administrators as group profits and reserves. Since these measurements are based on different and often conflicting goals and agendas, there is usually a tension between those who want to see one result versus another.

It is difficult for a medical group administrator to explain financial results to physicians, who generally have not had the training to understand financial statements and concepts (but neither have some group administrators.) For example, it is very difficult to explain that increasing overall group overhead or the percentage of overhead to revenue may be positive for group physicians. For example, if adding another business line at a 20 percent margin results in a higher overall group overhead but also an increase in physician income, it is a positive result for group physicians.

Medical groups need to agree upon generally-accepted standards and then measure those standards against organizational goals and objectives. Medical group administrators and managers should communicate financial results of group operations frequently and clearly to group physicians.

Notes

[1] "Information Systems," *Integrated Healthcare Report*, January 1995, p. 2.

[2] *Physician Practice Management Information Systems*, Volpe, Welty & Company, Jan. 3, 1995, pp. 68-69.

[3] Ibid., p. 70.

[4] *Ambulatory Care Management and Practice*, Edited by A. Barnett, M.D. and G. Mayer, RN, EdD, FAAN, p. 451.

[5] *Why Physicians in Group Practice Earn Less than Comparable Colleagues in Solo Practice*; a brief critical paper. Group Practice Management, Incorporated, Columbia, Mo., p. 11.

Conclusion

Hopefully, this discussion has been useful in developing a better understanding of the development and management of medical groups. It is a brief overview of some of the challenges medical group leaders face in our dynamic health care environment. As stated by Rick Wesslund of BDC Advisors in San Francisco, Calif., successful development and management of medical groups requires a combination of leadership, capital and time:

Key ingredients for success[1]	
Leadership	• Overcoming inertia • Providing catalyst for action • Management skills • Partnership focus • Shared decision making
Capital	• Planning and development • Physician growth and recruitment • Protection from risk • Facilities development and acquisition • Systems development and acquisition • Management recruitment
Time	• Develop common vision • Establish guiding principles • Allow significant time to plan and implement

The next few years should bring additional complexity and excitement for both medical group physicians and administrators. As Yogi Berra aptly put it: "The future ain't what it used to be."

Notes
[1] BDC Advisors, San Francisco, CA, 1993.

Appendices

Administrator and Medical Director Responsibilities

Medical group administrator's responsibilities:

- Overseeing the daily operations of the medical group and working with the line department heads to develop and refine the efficiency and effectiveness of each of the departments in order to promote excellent operational systems.
- Studying and understanding all programs and plans that have been adopted by the board of directors.
- Overseeing the preparation of operational budgets, ensuring that all operational budgetary elements are addressed in the group's overall budgetary process, and ensuring that appropriate accounting systems are in place to furnish data on all financial matters.
- Developing operational staff plans and directing the filling of all operational staff positions.
- Developing capital equipment plans for new programs and ongoing operations, and overseeing the acquisition of the necessary equipment.
- Developing operational space need plans for ongoing operations and new programs adopted by the board of directors.
- Observing daily operations and identifying areas where modifications of policies and procedures will improve patient care.
- Developing sound billing and data retrieval systems and overseeing the claims-processing and collection systems to ensure timely cash flow.

- Ensuring that claims, complaints, and inquiries from patients are handled courteously, capably, and promptly.
- By working through the line departments, ensuring the regular training of personnel so they develop the knowledge and skills needed to perform their jobs and encouraging individual employee development so that future needs of the group are adequately met.
- Evaluating the objectives of the group from an operational viewpoint and in light of the changing medical delivery environment, and making recommendations to the board of directors concerning changes that may be appropriate given the group's objectives.
- Reporting regularly to the board of directors regarding significant operational issues, including plans for change, staffing issues, and operational problems.
- Attending regular meetings of the board of directors and shareholders meetings and offering advice and recommendations concerning issues under consideration, particularly as they may affect operations.
- Representing the group as the administrative delegate at various community meetings where such representation is appropriate.
- Studying and negotiating agreements and contracts with health plans under which the group provides medical care, then advising the board of directors of the outcome of such negotiations and reporting any difficulties that the agreements or contracts may pose.
- Keeping current on all developments in the medical arena on local, state, and national levels, and educating physician leaders and staff so that they can proactively respond to the various threats and opportunities
- Performing such other management duties as may be assigned from time to time by the board of directors.

Medical group medical director's responsibilities

- Developing and implementing policies, plans, and procedures to achieve and maintain high professional standards.
- Ensuring that the organization and its physicians comply with all medically-relevant licensing and regulatory bodies.
- Keeping current on technical and medical advances and innovations that might be of value to the practice.

- Monitoring and evaluating quality assurance, utilization review, and risk management activities.
- Assuming a major advisory role in the organization's educational programs, including continuing education programs for physicians, nurses and other professional personnel.
- Ensuring adequate physician coverage to meet patient needs and assisting with the physician selection, recruiting, and retention activities of the organization.
- If nonphysician allied health care professionals are utilized in the practice, ensuring that their professional requirements are met and assisting in establishing their requisite protocols.
- Acting as principal liaison between the physician staff and the nonphysician administration and management.
- Facilitating professional and cordial relationships between the organization and other organizations such as HMOs and other payers.
- Establishing and maintaining relationships with outside physicians and provider groups, assisting in contracting for their services when advisable, and ensuring the quality of care of these outside providers.
- Providing regular input into the planning and resource allocation processes of the organization.
- Assisting in the monitoring and evaluation of all physician and allied health care professionals for performance, compensation, and other purposes.
- Interacting with and responding to patient surveys and grievances regarding quality of care.

Example of a Medical Group Implementation Plan

Office Consolidations:

- Merge physician practices
  - Transfer assets according to asset merger proposal
  - Arrange for assignment or renegotiation of physician office leases
  - Complete new property, facility and equipment purchases, leases and subleases
  - Commence construction, if any
  - Assign office space to group physicians
  - Finalize relocation schedule/timing
  - Complete space remodeling
  - Prepare for relocation of practices
    - Order stationery, forms
    - Prepare and mail out announcements
    - Prepare patient communications (signage, handouts, etc.)
    - Retain moving company
  - Develop office staff orientation and training
  - Relocate physicians and staff
  - Develop future sites
    - Target strategic sites for future offices
    - Develop criteria for new locations
- Develop procedure for transition of employees
  - Prepare a staff plan by location
  - Develop employee communication plan
  - Develop new job descriptions (as needed)
  - Prepare standard application and interview process

- Determine appropriate salary ranges
- Design orientation program
- Develop interview schedule
- Interview, hire and orient employees

Operations:

- Finalize governance and management
  - Elect board members
  - Appoint medical group officers
  - Define role of standing committees and appoint committee membership
  - Establish meeting schedules and locations
  - Finalize management team position descriptions
  - Recruit/select final management team
- Develop policies and procedures for office operations
  - Survey existing policies and procedures
  - Develop and implement policy manual
- Develop human resources program
  - Develop personnel policies
  - Develop and implement employee handbook
- Finalize physician/employee benefit package
  - Determine physician/employee benefit needs
    - Health, life, accidental death and disability, etc.
    - Retirement and deferred compensation plans
    - Malpractice insurance
- Solicit bids for plans/options
  - Review summary proposals with medical group
  - Select coverage/insurance providers/third party administrators
- Complete business licensure/setup
  - Fictitious/trade name registration
  - Local city licenses
  - Property tax filing
  - State and Federal tax identification numbers
  - Medicare and other providers numbers
  - Payer list
  - Logos, business cards, stationery, telephone numbers, etc.
- Develop medical records system
  - Develop initial medical records system
  - Evaluate long-term enhanced medical records systems
  - Develop long-term policies for charting, record storage, etc.

- Implement physician compensation system
  - Prepare compensation financial proformas for the current year
  - Implement productivity measurement systems
  - Develop compensation policies and procedures
  - Set-up tracking, reporting and payment mechanisms
- Develop annual budgeting systems
  - Design operating budgeting process
  - Design capital budgeting process
  - Develop first year operating budget and five year capital budget
- Develop physician database
  - Licensure
  - Continuing medical education
  - Board certification
  - Malpractice
  - Personnel information
- Set-up banking/fiscal systems
  - Evaluate/select banking service
  - Establish various accounts
  - Set-up lock box
  - Order check stock/supplies
- Set-up risk management program
  - Evaluate, select insurance carriers
  - Determine compliance with regulations (OSHA, etc.)
  - Standard medical records

Management Information Systems (MIS):

- Review existing physician office MIS systems
  - Develop transition plan using existing systems
  - Communicate transition plan to employees
- Establish criteria/specification for various areas for the medical group MIS system
  - Office operations
  - Claims processing
  - Billing and collections
  - Patient scheduling
  - Capitation management
  - Accounts payable and payroll
  - Financial reporting
  - Data reporting

- Recruit and select MIS consultant
- Evaluate available medical group MIS systems
- Solicit bids, select and implement medical group MIS system
- Develop financial systems
  - Set-up general ledger
  - Set-up accounts payable systems
  - Set-up billing and collection systems
  - Set-up financial reporting procedures
- Develop patient scheduling system
  - Survey current and competitive procedures
  - Identify vendors and solicit bids
  - Select and implement system
- Develop communications/phone system
  - Evaluate existing systems
  - Establish requirements for medical group
  - Evaluate and select options
  - Coordinate installation with facility planning

Managed Care Systems/Contracting/Marketing:

- Develop marketing program
  - Develop marketing objectives and strategy
  - Develop medical group identity program
  - Develop customer service program
  - Develop marketing materials
  - Print physician directory
  - Implement marketing program
- Develop managed care contracting strategy
- Develop physician panels
  - Define physician coverage requirements
  - Develop criteria for physician panel inclusion
  - Set-up/negotiate outside physician fee schedule
  - Develop utilization policy guidelines
  - Implement physician panels
- Identify ancillary services provided
- Identify hospital/other acute and subacute services provided
- Secure managed care contracts
  - Review existing managed care contracts
  - Implement managed care contracting strategy
    Initiate and conduct payer negotiations
  - Implement new managed care contracts

- Develop managed care systems and policies
  - Develop utilization review and quality assurance policies
  - Set-up case management systems
  - Develop managed care reporting systems
  - Develop physician incentive systems to manage risk